OXFORD MEDICAL PUBLICATIONS

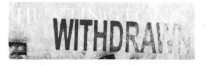

the**facts**

the**facts**
ALSO AVAILABLE IN THE SERIES

HUNTINGTON'S DISEASE

the**facts**

Oliver Quarrell
Clinical Geneticist
Sheffield Children's Hospital

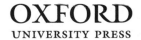

OXFORD
UNIVERSITY PRESS

OXFORD

UNIVERSITY PRESS

Great Clarendon Street, Oxford, OX2 6DP

Oxford University Press is a department of the University of Oxford.
It furthers the University's objective of excellence in research, scholarship,
and education by publishing worldwide in

Oxford New York

Athens Auckland Bangkok Bogotá Buenos Aires Calcutta
Cape Town Chennai Dares Salaam Delhi Florence Hong Kong Istanbul
Karachi Kuala Lumpur Madrid Melbourne Mexico City Mumbai
Nairobi Paris São Paulo Singapore Taipei Tokyo Toronto Warsaw

and associated companies in Berlin Ibadan

Oxford is a registered trade mark of Oxford University Press
in the UK and in certain other countries

Published in the United States
by Oxford University Press Inc., New York

© Oliver Quarrell, 1999

The moral rights of the author have been asserted

Database right Oxford University Press (maker)

First published 1999

A catalogue record for this book is available from the British Library

Library of Congress Cataloging in Publication Data
Quarrell, Oliver.
    Huntington's disease: the facts/Oliver Quarrell.
    (Oxford medical publications) (The facts)
    Includes index.
    1. Huntington's chorea Popular works.   I. Title.   II. Series.
III. Series: The facts (Oxford, England).
    [DNLM: 1. Huntington's Disease.   WL 390 Q13h 1999]
RC394.H85037   1999   616.8′51—dc21   99–31801
                    ISBN 0 19 262930 1 (Pbk)

Typeset by EXPO Holdings, Malaysia
Printed in Great Britain
on acid-free paper by
Biddles Ltd, Guildford & King's Lynn

Preface

Huntington's disease poses lots of problems. Whether you have Huntington's disease, are caring for someone with Huntington's disease, or are at risk of developing the condition in the future, you are likely to have lots of questions. You may see a number of different professionals from time to time. Some of the more obvious professionals involved include: your local family doctor, a neurologist, a clinical geneticist, and possibly a psychiatrist. In addition, other professionals such as social workers, speech therapists, physiotherapists, nurses, and home helps are likely to be involved with your family. You may also come into contact with a patients' organization, either to obtain information, or to donate money, or to attend meetings of local groups. You and your family may obtain help, support, and information from any or all of these sources at different times. One aim of this book is to supplement these various sources of information.

A second aim of this book is to give the reader a greater understanding of the problems involved in caring for relatives with Huntington's disease, even though the solutions to these problems may be difficult to find. The first part of the book, Chapters 1–3, discusses some of the main medical facts. It is important to emphasize that, although patients with Huntington's disease have features in common, not everyone shows every aspect of the condition. Some carers have more problems with the physical aspect of the disease, whilst other families have more difficulty with the mental and personality changes that can occur. While there is no treatment to stop nerve cells in the brain dying early, there are ways to help families cope with some of the problems that occur. It is frustrating for families to realize that there is no magic cure for Huntington's disease; but doctors too are frustrated by not having all the answers to problems.

Huntington's disease is a genetic condition. A third aim of this book is to explain how the identification of the gene has improved our knowledge and made available more options if you are at risk of developing Huntington's disease. Television programmes and newspapers frequently discuss the impact of genetic testing. Indeed, Huntington's disease is becoming more familiar to the general public, in part because of media stories, both factual and fictional. Chapter 4 concentrates on an explanation of the genetic aspects of the disorder and describes the story of the cloning of the gene. Nowadays, doctors offer genetic counselling to most families. Alternatively, the family may take the initiative and ask for genetic counselling. Chapter 5 describes various aspects of genetic counselling. It is important to remember that although you will always be offered genetic counselling, you do not have to attend straight away. It is perfectly acceptable to delay attending the genetic clinic until you are ready. Although you may discuss genetic tests with a counsellor, it is for you to decide if they are in your best interests.

A fourth aim of this little book is to consider prospects for the future. Chapter 7 describes the changes that occur in the brain; that leads on to a discussion of the latest research activity and ideas for future research.

Finally, patients' organizations play a prominent role in partnership with professionals, so Chapter 9 explains how these groups have developed in different countries.

Huntington's disease is a rare disorder and it is easy to think you are alone. In a town with a population of a quarter of a million, there will be approximately 18–25 patients diagnosed with Huntington's disease, but there will be many more people at risk of developing the condition, so it is a significant issue for a lot of people. The overall aim of this book is to give you more knowledge and understanding of Huntington's disease.

Sheffield
1999   O. Q.

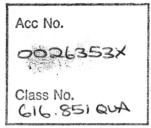

Acknowledgements

I would like to thank a number of people who have helped me during the preparation of this book. Firstly, I must acknowledge and thank my wife Gillian for her support and encouragement during this project. I am of course indebted to my teachers, but I have also been inspired by the families with Huntington's disease whom I have met over the last fifteen years. Although any errors or omissions are mine, I am grateful to Audrey Tyler, Sue Watkin, Cath Stanley, Nora Shannon, and David Craufurd for reading and checking all or parts of the manuscript. Gerrit Dommerholt of the International Huntington Association gave me information on the history of the development of patients' organizations and provided the list of addresses in the appendix. Finally, I would like to thank the staff of Oxford University Press for their help and support.

the**facts**

CONTENTS

Glossary

This glossary contains a list of some of the technical words used in this book. In some cases the definitions only refer to the way the word is being used in this book.

Affect—another term for a persons mood or emotional disposition.

Amniocentesis—the technique of removing fluid from around a baby at around the sixteenth week of pregnancy.

Antibody—a protein produced by the body in response to a foreign protein. The antibody binds to the foreign protein and helps with its removal. Antibodies are also used in scientific experiments to bind to specific proteins.

Autosome—any one of chromosomes 1–22. That is any of the non-sex chromosomes.

Autosomal dominant inheritance—a mutation or change in the DNA on one of the autosomes which is passed down from one generation to the next. The mutation dominates over the normal copy of the gene on the other autosome and causes a disease or condition to develop.

Axon—the long process of a nerve which transmits the impulse to the next neurone.

Basal ganglia—collection of nerve cells below the cortex of the brain. A number of different areas can be identified; those important to Huntington's disease include the caudate and putamen.

Bradykinesia—an abnormal slowness of movement.

Caudate—part of the basal ganglia which is especially affected by Huntington's disease.

Chorea—random purposeless involuntary move-ment.

Chorion biopsy—taking a small piece of the placenta or afterbirth during a pregnancy. This contains fetal cells which can be used for pre-natal diagnosis. It is also sometimes called chorionic villus sampling or CVS.

Chromosome—structure in the nucleus of a cell which contains a tightly coiled linear thread of DNA. With the exception of eggs and sperm every cell has 46 chromosomes. They are in pairs. Eggs and sperm contain only one chromosome from each pair and have 23 chromosomes.

Cognition—process involved in knowing and thinking but distinct from emotion.

Cognitive flexibility—ability to adapt plans and concentrate on more than one task.

Cognitive impairment—reduce ability to think.

Cortical—the outer layer. In this context it is the outer layer of nerve cells of the brain.

Cytoplasm—the area of the cell outside the nucleus.

DNA—an abbreviation of deoxyribonucleic acid. This is the chemical structure of the genetic material. It contains 4 types of nucleic acid: adenine, thymine, cytosine, and guanine (A, T, C, and G). These form the letters of the genetic code.

Delusions—false beliefs which are inconsistent with someone's knowledge or experience. Religious beliefs are excluded.

Dementia—loss of intellectual power usually as a result of an illness.

Disinhibition—being unrestrained by the usual social constraints on behaviour which could include anger, swearing, or inappropriate sexual advances.

Dystonia—prolonged contraction of muscles which results in the limbs, neck, or face adopting unusual positions.

Executive functions—those parts of the brain concerned with planning ahead.

Expanded polyglutamine tract—enlargement of the series of glutamine building blocks in the first part of the huntingtin protein.

GABA—one of the neurotransmitters in the nerve cells of the caudate and putamen basal ganglia. Nerve cells which use this neurotransmitter are particularly susceptible to Huntington's disease.

Glutamate—one of the neurotransmitters of the brain. In the context of Huntington's disease it is the neurotransmitter from nerve cells in the cortex to the caudate and putamen basal ganglia.

Glutamine—one of the building blocks of proteins. There is a series of glutamine building blocks in the first part of the huntingtin protein.

Histones—proteins around which the DNA molecule is wound to form a chromosome.

Huntingtin—the protein coded by the gene for Huntington's disease. The normal protein has a repeat series of less than 36 glutamines whereas abnormal huntingtin has more than 36 repeats of glutamine.

Linkage—two genes close together on the same chromosome so they are more likely to be inherited together.

Mania—a recognized psychiatric condition in which a person is very energetic and often has grandiose ideas such as having extreme wealth.

Marker—a variation in the DNA molecule close to a gene of interest, in this case Huntington's disease, such that the marker and the gene are usually inherited together.

Metabolize—the process of turning food into useful products for the body. In the context of Huntington's disease the word relates to the production of energy.

Mitochondria—specialized parts of the cell involved in the production of energy from fats and sugar.

Morbid jealousy—an unreasonable belief that a partner is being unfaithful.

Mutation—a change in the DNA molecule which results in a disease. In the case of Huntington's disease the mutation is an unstable expansion of a trinucleotide repeat.

Nerve cell body—the part of the nerve cell which does not include the projections for receiving or transmitting impulses.

Neuronal intranuclear inclusion—abnormal accumulation of the first part of the huntingtin protein and another protein called ubiquitin in the nucleus.

NII—abbreviation for neuronal intranuclear inclusion (see above).

NMDA—a subclass of glutamate receptor thought to be involved in Huntington's disease. (The abbreviation is for a chemical N-methyl-D-aspartate).

Nucleus—specialized part of a cell which contains the genetic material.

Penetrance (of a gene)—the proportion of people with a gene for a particular disease who actually develop the condition. In the case of Huntington's disease penetrance is nearly 100%.

Polyglutamine tract—section of the first part of the huntingtin protein which contains a repeated number of building blocks called glutamine.

Predictive test—a test undertaken on individuals at risk of Huntington's disease before the condition has started to see if they have inherited the gene.

Projection—the area of the nervous system to which impulses are transmitted from a particular group of nerve cells.

Putamen—part of the basal ganglia especially sensitive to Huntington's disease.

Remacemide—a drug which blocks NMDA receptors. Research is currently underway to see if it is effective for Huntington's disease patients.

Rigidity—stiffness of movement.

Subcortical—a general term for the nerve cells in the brain which are below the cortex.

Transgene—insertion of a gene of interest into another cell. If it is inserted into an egg cell which eventually becomes an animal, such as a laboratory mouse, then the animal is said to be transgenic.

Triplet—a three-letter code of the DNA molecule which specifies one of the building blocks of a protein.

Ubiquitin—a protein which is involved in the clearance of other proteins from cells.

Unstable expansion of a trinucleotide repeat—the nature of the mutation in Huntington's disease and several other disorders. It refers to the fact that the normal gene has a code for one of the building blocks (in the case of Huntington's disease the building block in question is glutamine) which is repeated a number of times. The abnormal gene has a much larger number of repeats. It is unstable because the number of repeats can vary when it is inherited by the next generation.

1
Facts and figures about Huntington's disease

What is Huntington's disease?

Huntington's disease is a condition which affects the brain. Our brains contain millions of nerve cells, each one of which makes connections with lots of other nerve cells. We use our brain for thinking, planning, and remembering events, but the brain also controls a lot of processes automatically. The brain controls movements of the body so that they are smooth and automatic. For example, when you wanted to pick up this book you were able to do so because your brain was able to co-ordinate a number of different functions without you giving each one any conscious thought. If we consider some of the steps in this example: information from your eye and where your hands were in relation to the book was co-ordinated; you could then smoothly move your arm so that your hand was close to the book and you could use your fingers and thumb to pick up the book. All this movement was achieved without unbalancing the rest of your body.

The nerve cells in particular parts of the brain serve specific functions. In a person with Huntington's disease some nerve cells, in specific areas of the brain, die back early. This produces a pattern of problems which allows doctors to make a diagnosis of Huntington's disease. We will consider this pattern of nerve cell loss in Chapter 6, but for the moment will continue with some of the more basic facts about Huntington's disease.

The history of Huntington's disease

Why is it called Huntington's disease?

Many medical conditions are named after the doctor who recognized and gave a clear description of the pattern of problems associated with a particular disorder. In our case Huntington's disease is named after an American doctor called George Huntington. Although George Huntington was not the first person to describe the condition, his was the first clear, succinct account. When other doctors then wanted to write about their patients they called the condition **Huntington's chorea**. This now raises two questions.

What is 'chorea' and why has the name been changed to Huntington's disease?

A lot of medical terms are derived from either the Greek or Latin languages. The word 'chorea' comes from the Greek word for 'dance'. Nowadays, it is a word used to describe unwanted, extra, involuntary movements. Some involuntary movements are useful, such as breathing and blinking, but a person with Huntington's disease has movements of the face, body, and limbs which are random and purposeless. I will describe the various types of movement problems in more detail in the next chapter. As chorea is not the only movement disorder which can occur in Huntington's disease, and as the emotional and behavioural aspects can be more of an issue for the patient and the family, the term **Huntington's disease** has become fashionable in recent times. As with any fashion it takes time for the change to be widely adopted so it is possible that you will still find some professionals using the term 'Huntington's chorea'.

What was so remarkable about George Huntington's description?

George Huntington wrote a medical paper which was published in the Philadelphia-based *Medical and Surgical Reporter* in 1872. The title of the paper was 'On Chorea'. Huntington's disease is not the only cause of chorea, and at that time chorea was often the result of an infection. Nowadays we seldom see chorea caused by infection, but that is another story. Most of George Huntington's paper was about the then most common cause of chorea. However, on the last page he described an hereditary form of chorea. His account of families with the hereditary form of chorea is very succinct and accurate, and it enabled other doctors to separate this cause of chorea from the others.

It may be interesting to take a slight diversion and comment on why George Huntington was in a position to know so much about Huntington's disease at such a young age. George's forebears migrated from England to the East Coast of America, and his father and grandfather practised medicine in an area of Long Island, New York. In this area they saw and looked after families with hereditary chorea. George first met someone with Huntington's disease at the age of eight, when he travelled on medical rounds with his father. Having qualified as a doctor, George wrote his paper soon afterwards, while still only 21 years old. He was able to draw on his father's experiences of the condition and the original manuscript contains notes made by his father.

Other landmarks in the history of Huntington's disease

In the early part of the twentieth century there were relatively few publications on Huntington's disease, but the pattern of inheritance was confirmed. In addition, there were attempts to identify the number of patients in a given geographical area, and some of the changes in the brain were documented. With time, these studies became more sophisticated. The first book dealing solely with Huntington's disease was published by Michael Hayden in 1981. The book was based on his study of Huntington's disease families in South Africa, but it is clear that most of the natural history, basic genetics, and patterns of nerve cell damage in the brain had been well established by that time.

Other notable landmarks include the foundation of a patients' organization, called the Committee to Combat Huntington's Disease, which was founded in the USA by Marjorie Guthrie in 1967. Her husband, the folk singer Woodie Guthrie, had died of the condition that year. The development of patients' organizations is described in more detail in Chapter 9.

The struggle to identify the problem with the gene which causes Huntington's disease covers the period from the 1980s to 1993 and will be described in Chapter 4, but for now I want to concentrate on the numbers of people affected and some aspects of the natural history of the disease.

How many people are affected?

In order to answer this question a doctor has to define an area which contains a large number of people, count the number of patients with Huntington's disease who were alive on a particular date, and compare that with the number of healthy people in that area who were alive at the same time. This seems simple enough, but there are a number of problems with this type of study. Defining a reasonable area is important; if the area is too small then the result can be very misleading. If we take a row of houses which contain 10 people and 1 person has Huntington's disease then 1 person in 10 has Huntington's disease—but this answer is absurd. If the area is too large, then it may be difficult to identify all the patients with Huntington's disease. The early studies tended to underestimate the number of Huntington's disease patients. If we look at some of the studies of numbers of patients in the UK, which have been done in the last twenty years or so, then it is clear that results ranged between 4 and 10 patients with Huntington's disease for every 100 000 of the population. Some studies were more sophisticated than others in the way they counted patients. These studies tended to give higher results so a convenient estimate is 10 patients per 100 000. This means that in the UK, which has a population of approximately 55 million, there are about 5500 patients with Huntington's disease at any one time. It is now easy to see that Huntington's disease is a rare disorder, but if we count the carers and close relatives of a patient then many more people are affected by Huntington's disease. In addition, a patient has Huntington's disease for a very long period of time, so the condition represents a significant problem.

Huntington's disease in various parts of the world

It is reasonable to ask if Huntington's disease occurs in all parts of the world and if different countries or continents have different numbers of Huntington's disease patients, and if so why? As we started with the UK it may be interesting to note that studies suggest very similar numbers of people are affected in European countries.

We can now go on to consider the English-speaking nations, since they were largely founded by migration from the UK and other parts of Europe. As might be expected the number of people affected by Huntington's disease is again in the range of 4–10 per 100 000 in Canada, the USA, and Australia. It is also interesting to ask if Huntington's disease affects the native populations. This type of information is more difficult to gather. It may be that there are fewer cases among these peoples, but detailed studies have not been undertaken. Similarly, studies of numbers of patients with Huntington's disease have not been undertaken in the Indian subcontinent; however, there has been a study of Huntington's disease among the immigrant population in the UK which gave a result of 1.75 per

100 000. There are a number of reasons why this figure could be an underestimate, so it is reasonable to assume that Huntington's disease does occur in India, and if it were possible to do a systematic study, the numbers of people affected could be similar to that seen in Europe. Detailed studies have not been undertaken in other parts of Asia with the exception of Japan, where it has been well documented that there are fewer cases.

Interesting things happen if relatively few people migrate to a sparsely populated part of the world. If one of the founders of that population has Huntington's disease and goes on to have a lot of descendants then the number of people affected with Huntington's disease can become unusually high. This has happened in Tasmania (Australia) and has also happened in an area of Venezuela. The large family which lives around the shores of Lake Maracaibo has been particularly important in the hunt for the Huntington's disease gene. This story will be told in more detail in Chapter 4.

When does Huntington's disease start?

This question gives the impression that the age of onset of Huntington's disease can be documented accurately. This is not so. A person does not go to bed healthy and wake up the next day with Huntington's disease. Many people at risk have asked me to describe how Huntington's disease starts. On the face of it, this is a reasonable question, but in fact it is difficult to give a clear answer. When doctors make a diagnosis of any condition they are effectively recognizing a pattern. The first subtle signs may be when someone starts to have mood changes or begins to be less tidy than they once were. This type of change can occur for many different reasons, apart from Huntington's disease. It is only possible to estimate that this must have been the start, when the more obvious signs, such as abnormal movements, occur later on. Someone experienced in seeing patients with Huntington's disease may be suspicious of changes in behaviour, and may recognize small abnormal movements as being chorea at an early stage, especially if there is a family history of the disorder. However, some of the early changes are very subtle, so an experienced professional may still want to see the patient again to be sure of the diagnosis.

However, most patients will not see an experienced doctor when they begin to have these very early symptoms, and it may be some years before the patient and members of their family recognize that there is a problem and seek medical help. If the doctor then asks 'How long have you had a problem?' the family will have some difficulty in remembering the start, because the condition has come on so slowly. They may be able to give an estimate of the start, but it will not really be accurate. For this reason the onset of Huntington's disease is best described as 'insidious'. As we will see in Chapters 4 and 5, the identification of the gene responsible for Huntington's disease has resulted in people at risk of developing it coming for **predictive tests** to see whether they will develop the disease p. 50–51 and p. 75–84). As someone who offers predictive testing, I sometimes see people who have very minimal chorea and am able to make a diagnosis much earlier than would have been likely a few years ago, before these tests were available. Before this, the patient and family would have waited much longer before seeing a doctor.

Despite these limitations, it has been possible to summarize the age of onset of patients in the form of a graph such as the one shown in Figure 1. Over the years there have been a number of studies estimating the age of onset of Huntington's disease, but they all result in an 'S'-shaped graph like this one. Given the shape of this graph, it is easy to work out that Huntington's disease can start at almost any age, but most people develop it between the ages of 35 and 55 years.

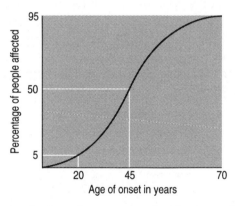

Figure 1. Age of onset curve for Huntington's disease. The age of onset curve is 'S'-shaped and indicates that the vast majority of people develop the condition before the age of 70 years. Only a few people develop Huntington's disease before or around the age of 20 years. The middle part of the curve is steep and reflects the fact that most people develop Huntington's disease between the ages of 35 and 55 years.

How long does Huntington's disease last?

Again, this is a very simple question but one which is difficult to answer accurately. In a study of patients with Huntington's disease in a particular area it is possible to know precisely when an affected relative died. The problem comes in trying to estimate when that person started with Huntington's disease. As we saw in the last section, it is possible to ask the family to give an estimate but it will not be absolutely precise. A number of studies have accepted this limitation and estimated the duration of the disease. The results have varied, but an average, of 15–16 years is a reasonable result. Of course you have to remember that this is only an average, so some patients will have had the condition for a longer and some for a shorter time. Given the difficulties of families accurately dating the onset of the condition I prefer to think of Huntington's disease as a condition which lasts around 20 years.

2
The physical features of Huntington's disease

As we saw in the last chapter, Huntington's disease lasts for a long time so it may be that you or your family can relate to only part of what is written here. In order to break up the story I have arbitrarily divided the description of a typical person into early, middle, and late stages. Let us first consider the problem of someone starting with Huntington's disease in middle age; we can then consider some of the features seen in people with particularly early onset or particularly late onset. Huntington's disease can start with either physical problems, changes in personality, or both. In some people the personality changes can occur well before neurological signs are obvious. However, in this chapter I want to concentrate on the physical aspects of the condition.

What are the physical signs in the early stages of Huntington's disease?

Some people are aware of Huntington's disease in the family and suspect problems early. On the other hand, as Huntington's disease develops slowly, some people may ignore or not notice problems for a very long time. One of the earliest physical signs of the disease is **chorea**—*involuntary movements*. It is very hard to explain the difference between chorea and someone who is fidgeting. When families ask me to point out what I am seeing I sometimes ask them to describe a particular colour, say, 'green'. As you might expect I often get the answer that grass is green. This allows me to go on and explain that most people cannot easily define 'green' but they have no difficulty in pointing out objects which are green. The same applies to the recognition of chorea by professionals and family members who have seen it regularly. In the early stages of the disease these extra movements occur infrequently and are not especially large. They are different from a fidgety movement, but I find it difficult to describe this in words. Chorea is usually considered as an involuntary movement, but patients with Huntington's disease also have problems with voluntary movement.

The problems with *voluntary movement* are often very subtle in the early stages of the disorder, and are best described as a slowing of movements. The technical term for this is **bradykinesia**. A doctor may specifically look for signs of slowing of movements by asking you to flick your eyes from one side to the other very rapidly. These eye movements are normally very rapid, but in someone with Huntington's disease it is possible to detect changes in the way they are performed. Other similar tests involve asking you to perform rapid alternating movements such as flicking the tongue from side to side or tapping their index finger and thumb together very rapidly. A doctor may also check the way you walk and may even ask you to take a number of steps putting the heel of one foot against the toe of the other (heel to toe walking). The speech of someone with Huntington's disease can be become slurred and for this reason a patient may be asked to repeat certain syllables, which can allow the doctor to detect subtle changes. It is important to realize that subtle changes in each of these tests can occur in a large number of conditions other than Huntington's disease but it is the *pattern* of abnormalities which allows a diagnosis to be made.

Surprisingly, these changes are often not experienced as major problems by the patient, although they clearly indicate that the disease has started. Many people are able to continue with their job for some time. It would be extremely unlikely that any drugs would be considered for the movement disorder at this stage. In fact, physical problems may be less important than difficulties with memory, emotion, or behaviour; these will be discussed in the next chapter. I have already made the point that the onset of Huntington's disease is insidious. Figure 2 shows the

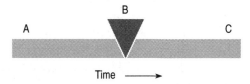

Time ⟶

Figure 2. Diagram showing the age of onset of Huntington's disease. During time period 'A' a doctor examining someone with a family history of Huntington's disease will say they are definitely unaffected. There is a variable time period 'B' when a doctor will be uncertain if the disease has started. Finally, if a doctor sees someone during time period 'C' there will be no doubt that the person is affected.

time course of the disease and time when you might seek medical help. Exactly what is said to a particular patient (or couple) will depend on when, during the course of the disease, you see a specialist and on what type of question you are asking. If you come and say that you think Huntington's disease has started, then it is relatively easy to answer you sympathetically but directly. On the other hand, I frequently see people in the clinic who show signs of the disease but who are completely unaware of them. If this is the case, it may be more appropriate for me to get to know these patients over a few appointments before voicing suspicions that the disease has actually started.

What happens after diagnosis?

Some families have complained to me that once a diagnosis of Huntington's disease is made they feel abandoned afterwards by the medical profession. I can understand how these feelings arise, since it may be that no specific treatment is required for a number of years. My own practice is to leave it up to the person or family concerned to decide whether they want to come to clinic once a year or wait until they feel it is necessary. An alternative to being seen in the clinic is to contact your own local doctor. In some countries, the patients' organization (which is discussed in more detail in Chapter 9) has a network of available contacts.

Another important point to come from this description is that if none of these signs are seen in people at risk of Huntington's disease they can be reassured that the disease has not yet started. Some people at risk are able to put the issue to the back of their minds whereas others look for signs of the disorder. It is important to realize that a doctor does not rely on one particular sign to make the diagnosis but on recognizing a pattern.

What about driving?

This can be a very sensitive issue for some people. In the UK the rule is clear: you have to inform the Driver Vehicle Licensing Authority (DVLA) if you have a medical condition which affects your fitness as a driver. There are several reasons why you may find this difficult: firstly, you have to have accepted the diagnosis in your own mind; and, secondly, it is difficult to contemplate the possible loss of easy mobility. Given that the features of Huntington's disease slowly worsen, it is almost inevitable that you will have to rely on someone else to drive you at some stage. The real difficulty is in deciding when this stage has been reached. It is often better if you inform the licensing authority yourself rather than getting into a position where this decision is forced on you. People who are in the early stages of the disease are sometimes given licences which can be reviewed on a regular basis.

What are the physical problems in the middle stages of the disease?

The term 'middle stages of the disease' is very imprecise, but it covers a long period of time where the condition has worsened so that the movement problems are obvious. If you are at this stage then you will probably no longer be working and will have difficulty performing household chores, but you will still have quite a lot of independence. For some people the diagnosis may not be made until this stage of the disease has been reached.

The chorea may be very obvious, with relatively large movements of the muscles of the limbs, face, and trunk. The slowing of movements will have worsened, but perhaps it will still be masked by the chorea. In addition, **dystonia** may become apparent. This term is used to describe abnormally slow and prolonged muscle contractions so that the limb, neck, or face involuntarily adopt unusual twisting positions. At this time there is a mixture of move-ment problems consisting of chorea, bradykinesia, and dystonia. Exactly what is seen in any one person depends on the exact mixture of these problems. Generally speaking, the chorea tends to plateau, but the bradykinesia and dystonia worsen. In some cases, as the disease progresses, the person appears stiff and **rigid**.

For some patients the movements are the main problem, but frequently the social, emotional, and behavioural problems are more of a concern to the family. At this stage patients may complain of problems with balance. Patients with Huntington's disease do fall, but I have always been more struck by the fact that the falls are relatively infre-quent, given that the choreic movements are so pronounced.

Drug treatment

It is possible to give drugs to slow down the move-ments, but this requires some thought. If drugs are given to reduce the chorea then it is likely that these same drugs will make the other movement dis-orders (bradykinesia and dystonia) worse. Drugs may need to be given to help with the patient's emotional and behavioural problems; but these drugs also have an effect on movement. A reasonable approach is to say that there is no medicine which will stop the nerve cells dying, but treatment is available to help with some of the problems this causes. A doctor, in discussion with the patient and the family, has to decide which is the main issue for everyone concerned and not treat the movements in isolation.

During this stage of the disease the patient's speech is likely to become more obviously slurred. In addition, difficulties with swallowing may also become apparent. These difficulties affect all aspects of the swallowing process, including taking an appropriate portion of food and chewing it fully. A referral to a speech therapist and a dietician can be useful to give advice to the carer about some practical issues, including how to deal with choking episodes.

What physical problems occur in the later stages of the disease?

Although this is arbitrary, I am assuming that the person with Huntington's disease has reached the stage of needing a lot of physical care, such as help with dressing, feeding, and going to the toilet. This care may be provided in an institution, such as a nursing home, or at home. If you are caring for someone at home then it is important to ensure that arrangements are made for you to care for yourself. You should not feel guilty for needing some time of your own. It may be that help from other family members is available. Unfortunately, the amount of professional help provided varies from place to place, but regular respite care may be a way forward. Behavioural difficulties often occur alongside physical problems, so getting the affected person to accept the need for respite care can be a real problem. In addition, respite care can be provided at home. Continuity of arrangements is important. My own practice is to encourage the involvement of social services early on so that support mechanisms are in place before a crisis develops. Whatever solution you reach, remember that as a carer you also need care and support; it may be that at this time you want to talk to other people in a similar situation, in which case you can attend meetings of the Huntington's Disease Association or other local support groups.

If the person with Huntington's disease is not very mobile, specially adapted chairs are available which help to prevent accidents due to the involuntary movements; one such is called the *Kirton*™ chair, as shown in Figure 3. A physiotherapist may be involved at this stage to give advice about trying to maintain the best posture so as to avoid problems in the future. Other adaptations to the home have to be considered. It is not easy to be specific because individual needs and circumstances vary, but practical solutions should be sought. This is when the advice of an occupational therapist can be particularly important.

There may be problems with incontinence. It should not be assumed that the incontinence is always due to Huntington's disease, so it is useful to check first that an infection is not present. However, in the majority of cases, practical solutions such as pads, closeness to the toilet, and regular toileting

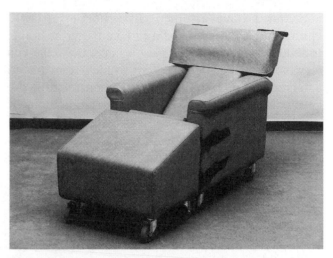

Figure 3. There are a number of special chairs available designed for someone in the later stages of the disease. The chairs are padded to protect the patient and are easy to keep clean. The leg-rest can be removed to help with mobility and care. In addition a sheepskin cover can be used to help pressure areas. (Photograph kindly supplied by Kirton Healthcare.)

have to be considered, as well as the use of easily removed clothes. Help and advice may be obtained from District Nursing Services.

A characteristic feature of Huntington's disease is weight loss. A proper explanation for this is not available, but it occurs in most patients. Part of the care may involve providing high calorie food supplements. Very occasionally feeding tubes are used, but the decision to use a feeding tube has to take into account the overall condition of the person with Huntington's disease and the wishes of the family.

So far I have assumed that the person with Huntington's disease is being looked after at home. Individual circumstances vary, so at some stage you may have to give some thought to long-term stay in a nursing home or similar establishment. Whilst the need to do this may eventually become obvious, it is not something which is done easily or lightly. If you have been caring for a loved one then it may be natural to feel a little guilty if and when the time for longer term care arises. Finding a suitable nursing home may not be easy, but the local support group may be able to give advice and information based on experience.

It has not been possible to describe all the practical problems which can occur or comment on possible solutions. However, Table 1 summarizes the role of the various professional and lay groups which may be involved in the care.

Table 1 Summary of agencies involved in the care of someone with Huntington's disease

Agency	Reason for involvement
Speech therapists, dieticians	Communication, swallowing problems, and nutrition
Occupational therapists, physiotherapists	Mobility, activities of daily living, and posture
District nurses	Incontinence and personal care
Social workers	Benefits and local care facilities, both respite and longer term
Family doctor	Relevant medication, support, and referral to other agencies
Local support groups	Support of the carer and information about local facilities
Specialist clinic	General support, relevant medication, and referral to other agencies

What are the differences if Huntington's disease occurs early in life?

Generally speaking, when Huntington's disease starts early in life, chorea is less prominent whereas slowness of movement and stiffness are more prominent. If you look at the age of onset curve on p. 9 you will see that occasionally Huntington's disease can start before the age of 20 years (and more rarely before the age of 10 years). This is called juvenile onset. There is no magic difference between onset at 19 and onset at 21–25 years, but it is still a useful definition for descriptive purposes. An early feature of juvenile onset is likely to be behavioural change and difficulty at school. Speech is likely to be slow and slurred. There may be a delay in establishing a diagnosis because the doctor may perceive the slow, stiff movements as less typical of Huntington's disease. Similar problems may occur if chorea is less prominent in an adult. When the disease starts in childhood, the rate at which movements become abnormal is faster than in the more usual mid-life onset. Epileptic fits occasionally occur in Huntington's disease, and when they do the person is more likely to be in the younger age range. Whilst the rate at which movement abnormalities develop may be faster than in a typical adult case, the duration of Huntington's disease is not dramatically different for children.

For a long time geneticists have noted that the affected parent of someone with juvenile onset is much more likely to be the father. I should hasten to emphasize that juvenile onset is still rare, so if a man is affected it does not follow that his children will necessarily have juvenile onset. Nonetheless, this statistical observation has needed an explanation; one is starting to emerge since the gene for Huntington's disease was identified and this point is discussed again on p. 54.

A problem can occur if the child of an affected father has behavioural problems but no obvious neurological signs. There is a temptation to use the genetic test on the grounds that if it is negative then the cause of the problem is something else (such as the child being disturbed by the effect of the illness in the family). Whilst this seems reasonable, most clinics dealing with Huntington's disease would be cautious because a positive result does not mean that behavioural problems on their own are due to Huntington's disease. They could have many causes, and for that child Huntington's disease may not be due to start for many more years. On the whole, it is better to wait until definite neurological signs are present and for the diagnosis to be more confident before using the genetic test.

What are the features when Huntington's disease starts late in life?

The other end of the spectrum from early onset is Huntington's disease starting late in life. As might be expected, the chorea tends to be more prominent and slowness and stiffness are less prominent. Superficially, the disease appears less disabling than when the onset is in mid-life or earlier. If Huntington's disease occurs late in life it is likely to be more difficult to establish a family history because the parents may have died many years previously, perhaps before they themselves showed signs of the condition. Chorea can be caused by conditions other than Huntington's disease, so the new genetic test has helped to resolve some difficult diagnoses. Not unreasonably, children of an elderly person with Huntington's disease may think that late age of onset runs in the family. Whilst there is some statistical evidence for this, it is not reliable enough to give practical information for the children, as we shall see in Chapter 4.

3
Behavioural and emotional aspects of Huntington's disease

A doctor or scientist giving a brief description of Huntington's disease will say it has three components: a **movement** disorder, impaired **cognition** (thinking), and a disturbance of **affect** (mood). The movement disorder was described in the last chapter; but now I want to concentrate on 'cognitive' or thinking problems and difficulties with 'affect' or mood.

We should not be surprised that behavioural and emotional problems, together with psychiatric illnesses are associated with Huntington's disease. The brain has a limited number of ways of coping with a variety of stresses. Nowadays there is much more openness about mental illness in newspapers and on television, and we know that many people become depressed, or mentally unwell, at some point in their lives. Someone with Huntington's disease has lost some nerve cells from the brain, so it is reasonable to suppose that one effect of this will be problems with behaviour and mental well-being.

I mentioned earlier that many families find it more difficult to cope with the wide range of behavioural and emotional problems than the physical aspects of the condition. If you are caring for someone with Huntington's disease you can find these problems often very frustrating. Since Huntington's disease lasts such a long time, and as each person is an individual, it is not possible to give a description that fits everybody. A further problem is that in some people it can be hard for their doctors and their carers to disentangle problems related to a depressed mood from those due to impaired thinking.

Some of what follows may be familiar to you from your experiences of Huntington's disease, but I want to emphasize that not everyone gets everything. Another important point to highlight is that the problems in Huntington's disease are *selective*. This theme of selective problems is taken up again in later chapters when we consider which nerve cells are damaged by Huntington's disease, but it is helpful to know that not all aspects of thinking are damaged.

What are the main problems?

The majority of carers to whom I have spoken recognize descriptions which include: irritability, outbursts of temper, and apathy. Other personality changes may occur, for example, the patient may become unusually tactless or thoughtless. These problems often disrupt family life and practical ways have to be found to get around the difficulties caused. In this chapter I have focused on the carer. As the disease progresses the patient is less aware of the effects of their behaviour on others. In my experience, it is usually the carer who complains about the behavioural and emotional problems.

When do these problems occur?

Changes in mood or behaviour may occur before the start of the clear-cut neurological signs. The changes may cause difficulties at work or difficulties maintaining the usual household chores. If mood and behaviour changes coincide with, or occur after, the neurological signs of Huntington's disease then it is not difficult to say that they are related to the condition. On the other hand, if they occur before neurological signs have become evident, then your doctor will have to keep an open mind as to whether or not Huntington's disease has started.

Can we explain the irritability and apathy further?

A brain has sometimes been likened to a computer. In many ways it is better than a computer because it can plan ahead, can switch between several tasks, and can cope with new information to change a plan. A simple example of switching between tasks would be preparing a meal whilst talking to the children about their activities at school. Similar situations occur at work, where it is possible to be doing a task whilst continuing a conversation with a colleague. Planning ahead is all very well, but it is frequently the case that during the day something occurs and new plans have to be made. These aspects of brain activity can be described as **executive functions** (planning ahead) and **cognitive**

flexibility (being able to concentrate on more than one task and to adapt your plans). It is these functions which are impaired in Huntington's disease. It may now be easier to understand why someone with Huntington's disease loses drive and initiative and in consequence appears apathetic. For the same reasons, the patient can become overloaded with tasks or have difficulty adapting to changing situations and respond with what seems to be unreasonable behaviour or an outburst of temper.

Trying to solve the problem is more difficult than describing it. A direct confrontation is unlikely to help, so other strategies have to be devised which include avoiding precipitating factors, avoiding the need to concentrate on several tasks at once, having some structure to the day, and encouraging the person to participate in joint activities for as long as possible. In general terms it is better to try these methods rather than immediately turning to drugs. Some of these problems can be explained by some of the changes which occur in the brain and these are discussed again in Chapter 6.

Appearance

Someone with Huntington's disease may well lose pride in their personal appearance which can lead to problems with washing, dressing, and shaving. Part of the problem may be related to apathy and part of the problem may be depressed mood. It is difficult to give specific advice on this except to try and encourage a routine without precipitating an outburst of temper. Again, telling someone with Huntington's disease to wash and dress is unlikely to work; although it can be more difficult, it is better to try gentle persuasion. If someone with Huntington's disease is living largely on their own, these problems may easily result in an unkempt appearance.

Sleep

Altered sleep patterns which result in someone with Huntington's disease being restless at night can be very disruptive of family life. Sleep disturbance may be a clue to the fact that someone is depressed. If this is the case then treating the depression may help. An alternative explanation is that a person with Huntington's disease may spend parts of the day dozing, and, as a result, may be restless during the night when the rest of the family are trying to sleep. If apathy and constant catnaps during the day are the problem then it may be a good idea to encourage the person to participate more in household activities.

Memory

In Huntington's disease, the memory does become impaired but it is not completely lost. This has been demonstrated in a number of psychological tests, which have shown that the results can be improved if the patient is given clues to aid memory. Obviously, as the disease progresses the problem worsens.

Although the term 'dementia' is medically correct, I have decided not to use this as a paragraph heading. This may seem surprising since the word dementia is easier to understand then the alternative of 'cognitive impairment'. This obviously reflects my own preference, but I want to stress that the problems seen in people with Huntington's disease are different from the more global difficulties seen in patients with Alzheimer's disease. We should not assume that a person with Huntington's disease has lost the ability to comprehend what is being said because of their appearance and speech difficulties. I want to return to this theme on p. 104 when considering some of the changes which take place in the brain.

Sexual problems

It is difficult to know the extent of sexual problems in families. In my own experience, loss of sex drive is extremely common; however, this is not the impression which is given in most medical articles.

Some years ago doctors published case reports and described the worst cases they had seen. This is understandable in the sense that we all remember unusual or striking cases. The problem with this approach is that it does not give a clear picture of what is happening with Huntington's disease families in general, compared with families without Huntington's disease. We can note that in his original paper, George Huntington described two married men with the disease, whose wives were living, who were constantly making love to some young lady or other. The point I want to make is that, as we all know, this behaviour may equally well be seen in men who do not have Huntington's disease.

Although loss of sex drive is usual, this is not always the case. A person with Huntington's disease may lose some of the social inhibitions which normally govern behaviour. This process is called **disinhibition**. We have all seen or experienced disinhibited behaviour associated with drinking too much alcohol. The result of disinhibition of someone with Huntington's disease can be sexual behaviour or remarks which are inappropriate at a particular time or place. This can be embarrassing to other members of the family, who may find it difficult to understand and control.

A person with Huntington's disease may think themselves less attractive and need reassurance. Occasionally, someone can falsely believe that their partner is having an affair. This is called **morbid jealousy**. If this occurs, then you may not be able to solve the problem by reassurance and may have to seek help, initially from your family doctor and then perhaps from a hospital clinic.

Which psychiatric illnesses can occur in Huntington's disease?

The answer to this question is 'almost any'. However, among the various psychiatric illnesses which can occur in Huntington's disease, the most common is depression. In some surveys of Huntington's disease, depression has occurred in about 40% of people. Unlike the movement disorder, this problem needs to be recognized and treated with medication. Whilst the movement disorder may be obvious to your doctor, signs of a depressed mood have to be actively sought. Someone with Huntington's disease may find it difficult to describe their feelings, but could well admit to lack of self esteem, feeling miserable, having difficulty with sleeping, a general loss of appetite, and a lack of interest in their usual activities.

Some people with severe depression can have false beliefs or **delusions**. One delusion was mentioned earlier in relation to morbid jealousy. Unlike schizophrenia, these delusions can be understood in terms of their depressed mood and feeling of unworthiness.

When we think of mood changes we most commonly think of depression but of course the opposite mood swing is **mania**. This means that the person is extremely active and rushes about undertaking a lot of projects in a very pressured way. If this happens then some very poor decisions can be made and a lot of money spent inadvisably.

Another well-known psychiatric disorder is **schizophrenia**. As may be expected, symptoms resembling schizophrenia occur in a percentage of people with Huntington's disease. These symptoms can be hearing voices or having false beliefs, for example, that people are spying on them or plotting against them. These symptoms need to be recognized and treated. The percentage of people with Huntington's disease who develop schizophrenia varies between studies, but up to 10% is a reasonable figure (of course, the other way of looking at this is that at least 90% do not).

Medication of psychiatric and behavioural problems

In the last chapter I stressed the need to avoid immediately turning to drugs to treat the movement disorder. In this chapter I want to indicate that whilst non-drug treatments should be tried first, psychiatric symptoms may well need to be treated with drugs. A side-effect of some of the treatments for psychiatric disorders is that they also slow down some of the choreic movements. I have decided not to give a list of the various types of drugs which are available but rather want to emphasize that treatments for depression and outbursts of temper are available and have improved in recent years. Many professionals who regularly see patients with Huntington's disease feel strongly that problems of depression and irritability should be treated and families not left to struggle on their own.

Is suicide associated with Huntington's disease?

Many studies have shown an increased rate of suicide in families with Huntington's disease compared with non-Huntington's disease families. Although suicides do occur, they are still rare events. In general terms, if someone with Huntington's disease is going to commit suicide then it is most likely to occur in the early stages of the disease.

Is alcohol a problem?

Many people with Huntington's disease find that a modest amount of alcohol has a more significant effect on them than previously. Indeed, people complain that neighbours mistakenly accuse them of being drunk because of the movement disorder.

Drinking excess alcohol will cause problems whether or not you have Huntington's disease. As problems with alcohol occur in the general population, so they also occur in people with Huntington's disease. As may be expected, if someone has a drink problem in addition to Huntington's disease then the behaviour problems are much worsened.

Conclusions

- Changes in personality and behaviour occur early in the course of the disease and can be present before the neurological problems begin.
- It is difficult to describe the full range of behaviour, but apathy, irritability, and outbursts of temper are common problems.
- A wide range of psychiatric problems occur in Huntington's disease of which depression is common and needs to be treated.
- These difficulties frequently cause more problems for a family than the movement disorder.
- There is no psychiatric illness or behaviour pattern which solely affects people with Huntington's disease. The same problems can occur in people who do not have the gene for Huntington's disease.

4

The genetics of Huntington's disease

Is Huntington's disease always inherited?

Huntington's disease is an inherited disease, passed on in the genes from one generation to the next. The genetic aspects of Huntington's disease were evident in George Huntington's description in 1872. We know that Huntington's disease can affect both males and females. We also know that if you are an affected parent with Huntington's disease, then when your children were born there was a 50% chance that they inherited the gene for the disease and a 50% chance that they did not. This requires an explanation.

Why do we have genes?

It may be useful to remember that your body is composed of millions of cells, and that these cells have specialist functions. Each cell contains a full complement of genetic material. The genes are the instructions for a cell to make proteins. Some proteins are present in every cell, whereas other proteins are only present in particular cell types. The proteins present in a liver cell will be different from those present in a muscle cell, and different again from those in a nerve cell of the brain. The different proteins allow the cell to grow and have specialized functions. Put very simply, a gene is the code for a particular protein. We could ask if different cells contain different genes but the answer to this is no. Each cell has two copies of every gene so it follows that in any particular cell a lot of genes are inactive.

Can we see individual genes?

Again the answer is 'no'. If you look at a cell under a microscope it is possible to see the genetic material within it packaged in the form of **chromosomes**. The chromosomes are seen most distinctly when the cell is about to divide.

Since each cell contains a full copy of the genetic material, it is possible to grow some cells from a blood sample in the laboratory and know that the chromosomes in these cells look the same as those present in other body cells. The chromosomes shown in Figure 4 came from one cell of a male individual. Essentially, the chromosomes were stained, which showed up a specific striped pattern, and then photographed. The chromosomes were cut out of the photograph, lined up in pairs according to size and staining pattern, and re-photographed. Nowadays, these steps are done with a computer program. It is clear that each cell has 46 chromosomes and that they are in 23 pairs. The chromosomes in the first 22 pairs are equal and these are

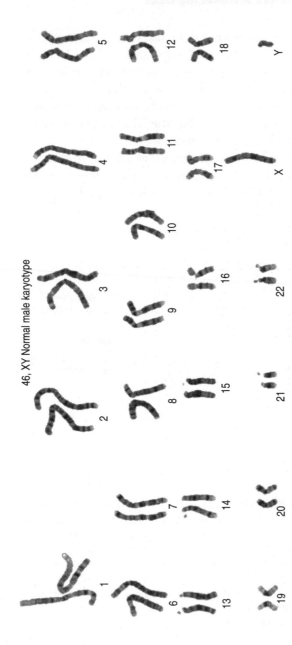

Figure 4. Photograph of the chromosomes from a single cell. The chromosomes are in pairs and are arranged in order of size. The last pair are called the sex chromosomes. In this case there is an X and a Y so the cell came from a male. (Photo courtesy of Mr M. Dyson.)

46, XY Normal male karyotype

called the **autosomes**. The last pair of chromosomes in this cell are unequal; they are the X and Y chromosomes which indicates that this cell came from a male. A cell from a female would have two X chromosomes. The last pair of chromosomes are called the sex chromosomes, but they do not feature in the story of Huntington's disease.

If we cannot see the genes, where are they on the chromosome? The answer is that a chromosome consists of a DNA molecule which is coiled up very

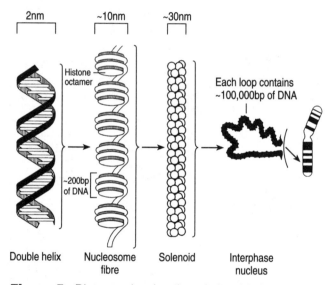

Figure 5. Diagram showing the relationship between DNA and a chromosome. The DNA molecule is wound on to proteins called 'histones'. Coiling the DNA in this way is like putting it around cotton reels. The DNA can be coiled again and again until the chromosome structure has been achieved. A gene is a stretch of the DNA molecule. Whilst it is possible to see the chromosome down the microscope it is impossible to see the individual genes this way.

tightly. Figure 5 shows a tiny section of a chromo-some in which a tiny part of the DNA molecule is unwound. A gene is a section of a DNA molecule which contains the message to make a particular protein.

How does a gene code for a protein?

The DNA molecule consists of two strings of chemicals which are usually called by the letters 'A', 'C', 'G', and 'T' after the first letter of their chemical name: 'A' for adenine, 'C' for cytosine, 'G' for guanine, and 'T' for thymine. A very tiny section of the DNA molecule can be represented by these letters, as shown in Figure 6. A DNA molecule can always copy itself because A always pairs with T, and C always pairs with G. Most of the DNA molecule does not code for anything, but, at particular points, sections of the DNA molecule code for the building

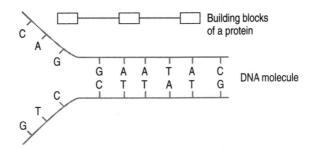

Figure 6. The DNA molecule consists of a double helix. There are rules for the way the letters are arranged 'A' always pairs with 'T' and 'C' pairs with 'G'. In a stretch of DNA which is a gene, three letters code for one of the building blocks of a protein.

blocks of protein. Sections of the DNA molecule which code for proteins are called genes. Within a gene, a group of three letters, say 'CAG', codes for one of the building blocks of a protein; another group of three letters, say 'GAA', codes for a different building block of a protein. A group of three letters which codes for a protein building block is called a **triplet**.

What about eggs and sperm?

It is often said that we have two copies of our genes and we inherit half our genes from our mother and half from our father. It is easy to see that when an egg is made (before it is fertilized) it contains one chromosome 1, one chromosome 2, one chromosome 3, etc., and, since eggs are made by females, one X chromosome. Similarly, a sperm contains one chromosome 1, one chromosome 2, one chromosome 3, etc., and, since sperm are made by males, it will contain either an X chromosome or a Y chromosome. In this way, when an egg and sperm fuse, the new cell or future child has two copies of each gene, half from the father and half from the mother. If the sperm contained an X chromosome, the future child will be a girl, and if it contained a Y chromosome, the future child will be a boy (see Figure 7). (This is a point which was lost on King Henry VIII.)

What is the pattern of inheritance in Huntington's disease?

It is fundamental to our understanding of Huntington's disease to realize that mistakes or errors can

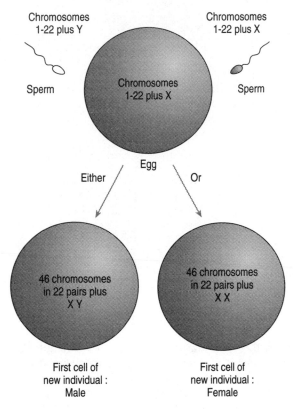

Chromosomes
1-22 plus Y

Chromosomes
1-22 plus X

Sperm

Chromosomes
1-22 plus X

Sperm

Egg

Either

Or

46 chromosomes
in 22 pairs plus
X Y

46 chromosomes
in 22 pairs plus
X X

First cell of
new individual :
Male

First cell of
new individual :
Female

Figure 7. Diagram to show that the sex of the baby is determined by the sperm (see text for an explanation).

arise in genes. I do not want you to think that in some way we are picking on Huntington's disease families: everyone has mistakes or errors in their genes. The technical term for errors in genes is **mutation**. As we have two copies of our genes this does not usually matter because the normal copy overrides the mistake. Unfortunately, the error in the Huntington's disease gene dominates over the

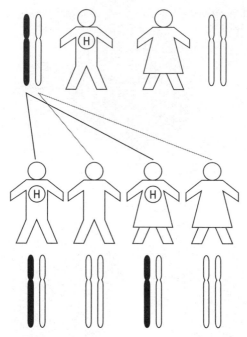

Figure 8. The pattern of inheritance of Huntington's disease. In this diagram the father has the Huntington's disease gene; he has a chromosome 4 with the Huntington's disease gene and a normal chromosome 4. Each parent gives a chromosome 4 to the children. The children are bound to get a chromosome 4 from the mother but it is 50:50 whether they get the chromosome 4 with Huntington's disease or the normal one from the father. It makes no difference whether the children are boys or girls.

The diagram could be redrawn with the mother having the Huntington's disease gene and the father unaffected. The effect for the children would be exactly the same; the chance of them inheriting the Huntington's disease gene would still be 50:50 and it would make no difference whether they were boys or girls.

normal copy and causes a problem. The gene for Huntington's disease is located on chromosome 4 (I will give a further explanation of this below), which is one of the autosomes; that is, a chromosome common to both sexes. Hence the pattern of inheritance of Huntington's disease is described as **autosomal dominant inheritance**. Since the sex of the child is determined by the X or Y chromosome in the sperm, it is clear that Huntington's disease can affect males or females equally, as shown in Figure 8.

Why do errors arise?

I am asked this question sometimes. The answer is that copying the genetic material is a complex process, so mutations occasionally occur. Not all mutations are detrimental. If a mutation occurs which allows a plant or animal a better chance of survival *and* reproducing then that gene will become more frequent in the population. It is this process which enables animals and plants to adapt and evolve. Some mutations are useful, the majority are neutral and just cause variations in the DNA molecule, and some, of course, cause disease.

How do we know the Huntington's disease is on chromosome 4?

I have included this section for interest, but, as it is a potted history of the discovery of the gene, you can skip over this section if you want to. The story starts back in the nineteenth century with Gregor Mendel and his peas. Gregor Mendel was an Austrian monk who worked out some laws of genetic inheritance from his work growing different varieties of peas in his monastery garden. He discovered that one copy of each gene pair is transmitted during reproduction, and that the different gene pairs are inherited independently of one another. Most of this is correct, but of course Mendel was not aware that genes are packaged on chromosomes. When eggs and sperm are forming, an interesting thing happens to the chromosomes, as shown in Figure 9. The chromosome pairs cross-over and exchange genetic material. If gene pairs are far apart on the same chromosome, or are on completely separate chromosomes, then they will be inherited independently. However, if they are close

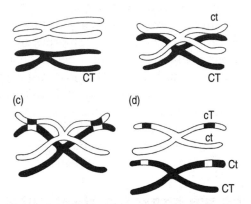

Figure 9. Diagram showing how genetic material is exchanged between chromosomes before eggs and sperm are formed. The letters cC tT represent different forms of 2 genes. Before eggs and sperm form the chromosome pairs double but do not completely separate, as in (a). They then come together in their pairs, as shown in (b). Genetic material is exchanged between the chromosome pairs (c), and then they separate as in (d). In this way the genetic material on the chromosome pairs is shuffled and one of the resulting chromosomes goes into either the egg or the sperm.

together on the same chromosome, then it is less likely that they will be separated by a cross-over, in which case they will be inherited together far more often than we would expect. The technical term for gene pairs close together on the same chromosome is **linkage**. The concept of linkage is not new; it was described in the early years of this century. Linkage was first described in humans in 1937 by two British geneticists Julia Bell and J.B.S. Haldane. They described the fact that the genes for haemophilia and colour blindness were close together on the X chromosomes, but at the end of their paper they commented that it would be useful to find a **marker** close to the Huntington's disease gene. In this context, a marker is a detectable genetic variation very close to the Huntington's disease gene. The marker has nothing to do with Huntington's disease other than being close to it on the same chromosome. In the case of haemophilia and colour blindness it is crucially important to realize that not all individuals with haemophilia are colour blind; but rather that if the two conditions occur together they tend to stay together because the genes are next door to each other on the X chromosome.

If the concept of linkage is not new, then why did it take from 1937 until 1983 to discover that the gene for Huntington's disease is located on the tip of chromosome 4? The first point to make is that, in large affected families, the gene for Huntington's disease and the genes for blood groups are inherited independently. This means that the Huntington's disease gene is not located close to a gene for blood group; therefore, blood groups are not useful markers for the Huntington's disease gene.

In order to locate the gene, several resources and techniques needed to come together. One resource was large families with lots of affected relatives alive. Such families are rare, but one very large family was known to exist in Venezuela, and blood samples were collected from this family. The other technique which was needed was the ability to detect some of the natural variations which occur in the DNA molecule. James Gusella and his colleagues worked to see if the gene for Huntington's disease was close to one of these natural variations in the DNA of the Venezuelan family and one other large family. They were successful in identifying that the gene for Huntington's disease was close to one of these variations, and since the particular variation was at the tip of chromosome 4 it followed that the gene for Huntington's disease was also located at the same place.

This work was published in November 1983 and sparked a whole new line of enquiry. The first step was to discover if the gene for Huntington's disease was on chromosome 4 in all families. Several researchers, from different countries, tested their families and concluded that 'yes' the mutation (or error) was on chromosome 4 in all families. This work took approximately two years, from 1984 to 1986. It was immediately realized that if the marker could be followed in a particular family, then unaffected offspring could be told whether or not they would develop Huntington's disease, depending on which form of the marker they had inherited (see Figure 10). The issue of predictive testing is considered in more detail in the next chapter. For the moment, it is enough to say that guidelines were developed at this time so that predictive testing was introduced in a carefully considered and controlled way.

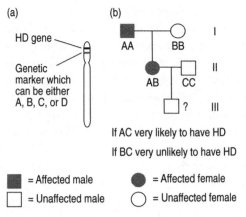

(a)

HD gene

Genetic
marker which
can be either
A, B, C, or D

(b)

If AC very likely to have HD

If BC very unlikely to have HD

■ = Affected male   ● = Affected female

□ = Unaffected male   ○ = Unaffected female

Figure 10. Diagram showing a predictive test using linkage. This test takes advantage of the fact that a marker (or natural variation in the DNA molecule) was found which was very close to the Huntington's disease gene (a). The genetic marker occurs in several forms. In any one individual the form of the marker next to the Huntington's disease gene was unlikely to be shuffled when eggs and sperm form. By following a marker through a family as in (b) a prediction could be made. The mother in generation II has inherited Huntington's disease and marker A from her father. Marker A is not present in her husband so a prediction can be made for her son. This type of test is cumbersome and relies on a family study.

Predictive tests based on linkage studies were used from 1986 until 1993. It is not necessary to discuss the technical aspects of this type of testing because the actual mutation in the gene was identified in 1993 and this has replaced the older test.

Why did it take 10 years to identify the gene?

It is easy to look back and wonder why it took so long. The technology to identify a gene improved over the 10-year period. The basic idea was that if one marker could be found which was close to the gene, then other markers from the same region might be even closer. As a chromosome is a length of DNA, it was very important to know if the gene was closer to the tip or the other side of the marker. It was soon realized that the gene was closer to the tip; but it was not until many more sections of DNA had been identified that the precise location of the gene was known. It was then a case of identifying the genes in a very tiny area to see if one contained a mutation. The mutation was eventually found in a gene called IT15. This is an odd name, but it represents the laboratory name for one of the fragments of DNA from the critical area of chromosome 4. Once the gene was identified it was possible to identify the protein for which it was coding. This protein had not been recognized before and was named **huntingtin**.

What is the mutation?

Genes are divided into sections, and it was realized that in patients with Huntington's disease the first section was larger than normal. The size of the normal gene varies a little, but Huntington's disease genes are always large. This can be explained by looking at the exact sequence of coding letters from the start of the gene.

The code for one of the building blocks of huntingtin is repeated a number of times in normal genes. This code is CAG. So normal DNA has the code: CAGCAGCAGCAGCAG, etc. The number of times CAG is repeated on a normal gene varies, but it is often about 15 to 20 times. A section of the DNA molecule which looks like this is sometimes

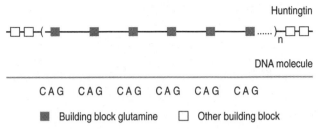

Figure 11. Diagram to show that repeating the DNA code CAG results in a protein which contains a string of the same type of building block, called glutamine.

called a **triplet repeat**; the triplet in this case being CAG.

The building block of the protein coded by CAG is **glutamine**, so it follows that the first part of the huntingtin protein contains glutamine repeated a number of times, as shown in Figure 11. As we have seen earlier, many terms in medicine and science are derived from the Greek and Latin languages. The Greek word for many is 'poly'; so this part of the protein is sometimes called a **polyglutamine tract**.

In someone with Huntington's disease, the number of CAG repeats is 36 or more. If there are 36 or more repeats, then the abnormal huntingtin protein will have 36 or more glutamines. The abnormal huntingtin protein has an **expanded polyglutamine tract** (Figure 12)

It is now a relatively simple laboratory procedure to check the number of CAG repeats from a sample of a person's cells. For convenience, we most often use some of the cells in a blood sample. You have to remember that, apart from eggs and sperm, each cell has two chromosome 4s, so we get two results from each individual. If someone does not have Hunting-

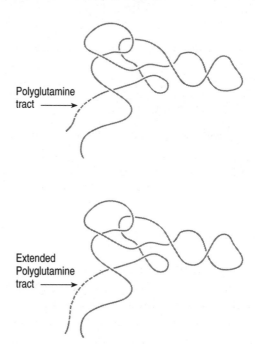

Polyglutamine tract ⟶

Extended Polyglutamine tract ⟶

Figure 12. Diagram showing the expanded polyglutamine tract in huntingtin.

ton's disease, then both copies of the gene will contain CAG repeats in the normal size range. However, if someone does have Huntington's disease, then one copy of the gene will be in the normal size range and the other copy will be in the Huntington's disease size range.

How does the laboratory test work?

The essential steps in the process are that when a blood sample is received the DNA is extracted. This

DNA is then treated so that only the CAG repeat portion on chromosome 4 is amplified many times. The size of the DNA fragment which has been amplified is totally dependent on the number of CAG repeats that are present. The more CAG repeats that are present, the larger the fragment. The next step is to measure the size of the fragments. This is done by loading the amplified DNA on to a gel and applying an electric current. The DNA molecule will always travel down the gel towards the positive terminal. Small DNA fragments travel down the gel faster than larger ones. After a given time, the gel can be stained and the size of the fragments assessed by the distance they have travelled. Figure 13 shows the results from one gel. The dark bands represent the amplified fragment containing the CAG repeats. It is possible to calculate how many repeats were present in each gene. Although Huntington's disease is not the only condition caused by the general mechanism of an expansion of a trinucleotide repeat in a gene, the scientific design of the test only amplifies the CAG repeat in the Huntington's disease gene.

Is there any overlap between the normal and Huntington's disease size ranges?

The direct answer to this is that there is a small overlap. It is possible for someone in the general population to have a gene with 36 or even 37 and 38 repeats and still be normal. You can see from Figure 13 that the overlap between Huntington's

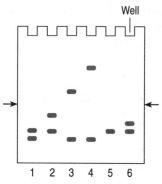

Figure 13. Diagram showing the results of an experiment to determine the size of DNA fragments containing the CAG repeat from six individuals. DNA from each individual was loaded into one of the wells at the top of the gel and an electric current applied. Larger fragments which contain a lot of CAG repeats do not travel as fast as smaller fragments. The gel can be stained to reveal the position of the fragments, in this case represented by dark bands. By knowing where different sized bands travel on a gel a scientist can know how many CAG repeats were present in each fragment. The *arrows* mark the position where a band containing 36 repeats would appear. As we have two chromosome 4s most people have two bands. In this diagram individuals 3 and 4 have one normal and one large-sized fragment and therefore have the gene. Individual 5 has only one band because both chromosome 4s had the same number of CAG repeats. In this diagram individuals 1,2,5, and 6 have CAG repeat sizes in the normal range and do not have the gene.

disease genes and normal genes does not occur very often. The fact that this overlap exists is usually mentioned in the genetic counselling for a predictive test, but this is considered again in the next chapter.

Is there any relationship between the size of the repeat and the age of onset of Huntington's disease?

The answer to this is 'yes'. In general terms, the larger the number of repeats the earlier the age of onset. This effect is most obvious for those with juvenile onset. People who develop Huntington's disease at a young age have extremely large numbers of repeats. For the more usual Huntington's disease repeat sizes shown in Figure 14 there is a very large range in the age of onset. This means that it is not possible to predict from a laboratory result when a particular patient developed Huntington's disease. This is even more important in the context of a predictive test because it is not possible to say when a person with a positive result will develop Huntington's disease.

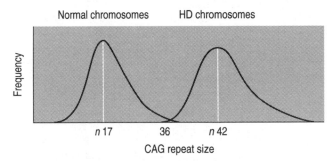

Figure 14. Diagram showing the small overlap between the size range of normal chromosomes and Huntington's disease chromosomes. The vast majority of normal chromosomes have less than 36 repeats. A common size is around 17 repeats. Huntington's disease chromosomes have 36 or more repeats. A common result is around 42 repeats.

Can we explain why most juvenile cases have affected fathers?

It has been noted since 1969 that in cases of juvenile onset Huntington's disease the affected parent is most likely to be the father. It is now possible to explain this observation. If we consider a person with two genes with normal sized repeats, say 17 repeats, on one gene and 20 repeats on the other then the vast majority of eggs or sperm will have either a gene with 17 repeats or 20 repeats. There may be the odd egg or sperm with 16 repeats or 18 repeats but these are very rare. On the whole,

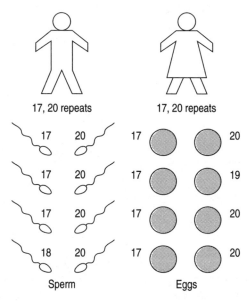

Figure 15. Diagram to show stable inheritance of normal size CAG repeats in males and females. Only the odd egg or sperm contains a change from one of the original sizes.

transmission of the repeat size down the generations is reasonably *stable* (Figure 15).

By contrast, repeat sizes in the Huntington's disease range are *unstable* when transmitted down the generations. Although repeat sizes can increase or decrease in eggs and sperm, the general tendency is for them to become larger. The tendency for repeat sizes to increase is much greater in sperm than in eggs. This is shown in Figure 16. A man

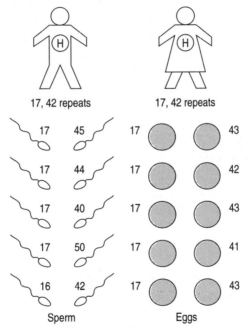

17, 42 repeats   17, 42 repeats

Sperm		Eggs	
17	45	17	43
17	44	17	42
17	40	17	43
17	50	17	41
16	42	17	43

Figure 16. Diagram to show the unstable inheritance of CAG repeats in the Huntington's disease range. The Huntington's disease genes in the eggs and sperm are usually around the same size as the parent, but in the case of a male an occasional sperm will have a very large increase in size.

affected with Huntington's disease has basically two types of sperm: those with the normal-size copy of the gene and those with the Huntington's-disease-size copy. The sperm with the normal-sized copy of the gene will be as stable as before, but there will be considerable variation in the number of repeats in those sperm that contain the Huntington's disease gene. Very occasionally a sperm can form with a very large increase in the number of repeats. Although there is some variation of repeat size in eggs, such very large increases do not occur. Now that we know that differences occur in repeat sizes between eggs and sperm it is easy to understand why most cases of juvenile onset have inherited their gene from their father. You should not worry about this too much if the affected person in your family is male because very young onset is rare.

Some scientists summarize the nature of the Huntington's disease mutation by calling it an **unstable expansion of a trinucleotide repeat**. At first sight this seems very technical; however, given the explanations in the previous few sections I hope you can see that this is actually a neat summary of the mutation.

Can new mutations occur in Huntington's disease?

Before 1993 the answer to this question would probably have been 'not really'. It was long held that new mutations were exceptionally rare. It was not unknown for someone to have Huntington's disease and for their parents to be unaffected; but this was often dismissed by saying there could have been non-paternity; or that one of the parents could have died from other causes before they developed Huntington's disease. However, now that we understand what is wrong with the gene, it has become easier to prove how new mutations arise.

Some people in the population have a normal gene with a repeat number in the high 20s and low 30s. As they have less than 36 repeats they do not develop Huntington's disease. In the vast majority of cases the gene is transmitted to their children without any increase in size, but just occasionally a man with this type of normal gene can produce a sperm which has a repeat size in the Huntington's disease range. If this happens then a new mutation has started. In some genetic disorders new mutations tend to arise in sperm, and Huntington's disease can also be added to that list.

Does everyone with more than 36 repeats develop Huntington's disease?

In an earlier section I mentioned the occasional overlap between the size of normal genes and those which cause Huntington's disease, but there is also a second complication to the issue of the lower size of Huntington's disease genes.

Before the gene was identified, doctors were clear that if someone inherited the gene they would develop Huntington's disease, provided they lived long enough. The technical term for this is that Huntington's disease is **fully penetrant**. Not all genetic conditions show full penetrance. It is possible for someone to have inherited a gene which causes a disease, not be affected themselves, but pass the gene to a child who is then affected. When this happens the disease in question is described as showing **incomplete penetrance**.

In exceptional cases someone with a family history of Huntington's disease and 36–39 repeats may live to an old age and die before showing signs of the disease. At this time it is not possible to give any precise information on how often this can happen. It may be better to describe Huntington's disease as **almost fully penetrant** to take account of the rare exceptional case. Unfortunately, not all people with 36–39 repeats develop Huntington's disease late in life, so it is still not possible to give an indication of the age of onset if a predictive test is positive.

5

Genetic counselling

If you, or a member of your family, has Huntington's disease then you will be offered genetic counselling. The offer may come from a hospital specialist around the time of diagnosis. Alternatively, you may initiate the referral yourself by asking your local doctor to refer you to the genetic clinic so that your questions can be answered. This could happen when a relative tells you that Huntington's disease is in the family; or it may be that, despite having known the family history for some time, you now judge that it is appropriate to get further information. Depending on your circumstances, you may go along to the genetic clinic as an individual, or more likely attend with your partner and have discussions as a couple.

The purpose of this chapter is to describe what is involved in genetic counselling and the options available to you.

Who are genetic counsellors and where do they work?

Usually, medical doctors lead genetic counselling teams. They are specially trained to give information about genetic disorders and to explain the implications of genetic tests. The genetic tests are performed by scientific staff in the laboratory. It is unlikely that you will meet the scientists involved in analysing genetic tests of your family, but there are other members of the team with whom you may have a great deal of contact. These are non-medical genetic counsellors who have a background in nursing or related disciplines, and are able to provide additional help and support.

Genetic conditions are rare, so genetic teams are usually based at large hospitals, and serve a population of 2–4 million people. This does not necessarily mean that you will have to travel to the large hospital, because the genetic teams hold clinics at the local hospitals at regular intervals.

What is genetic counselling?

The main purpose of genetic counselling is to provide information about Huntington's disease (or, for that matter, other genetic disorders), so that individuals or couples may make informed choices. Genetic counselling should be considered as a *process*, which suggests that the information-giving may take place over a period of time. It is reasonable to ask: 'How does genetic counselling differ from any other medical consultation?' Many medical consultations involve the doctor giving advice or recommending a particular form of treatment; whereas genetic counselling involves discussing options with you and then allowing you to decide which is the best way forward. It is not good enough to simply give information to people and say: 'Well these are your options; now you choose'. The doctor or counsellor has to understand your particular circumstances and support you in a way that allows you to make your own decisions. Geneticists describe the process as 'non-directive' and 'non-judgmental'; this emphasizes the point that you are not told what to do. These general principles underlie all genetic counselling sessions, although each genetic counsellor has an individual style.

An essential step in any genetic counselling process is the construction of a diagram of your family tree such as the one shown in Figure 17. One reason for drawing the family tree is to provide an easy record of your family history. It also helps to illustrate the point that we all share genes with our relatives. Genetic counselling also differs from other forms of medical consultation, in that it is concerned with the whole family: parents, children, aunts, grandparents, uncles, and cousins. This is described as the extended family or the kindred. You may be very concerned if a member of your family has, say, high blood pressure, but it does not have a direct bearing on your own health. However, a diagnosis of Huntington's disease has implications for you and all your close relatives.

What about confidentiality?

You may worry whether your details will remain confidential if other members of your family attend the same clinic. Genetic consultations are as confidential as other medical visits. Members of the genetic staff will not talk about you to other family members and vice versa. Of course, this does not stop you talking about your consultation with anyone you choose.

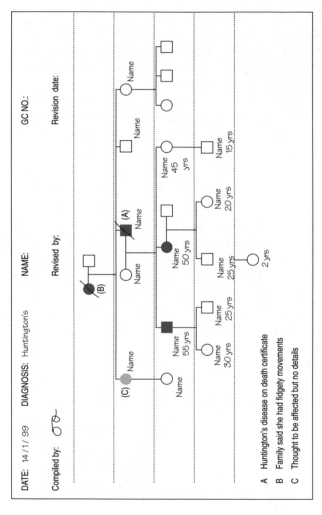

Figure 17. A family tree. This type of diagram is constructed by most genetic clinics and helps with the discussion of the illness in the family. Males are represented as squares and females as circles. Filled circles and squares represent those who have or had Huntington's disease. A line through the symbol indicates that the person has died.

When will we go for genetic counselling?

Members of a family will be told that genetic counselling is available. Some members of a family will take up the offer straight away, while others may wait some time before coming forward. As genetic counselling is about giving information and helping you to make your own decisions, it cannot be imposed by anyone else. The best time for the counselling team to see you in the genetic clinic is when you request it. This may seem obvious, but occasionally family doctors or specialists send people for genetic counselling at a time when they are not yet ready for it. When this happens the genetic counselling session is usually unhelpful for all concerned.

Who needs genetic counselling?

The simplest answer is that anyone concerned about the risks of developing or passing on Huntington's disease can benefit from genetic counselling. The person or couple who want information should attend the clinic; it is they who have to make the right choices for themselves. You do not know all the issues of concern to an adult child, brother, sister, or even your partner, so you cannot attend the clinic on their behalf. They need to attend a counselling session in their own right to express their own concerns and ask their own questions. In practice we can identify several different groups who come for genetic counselling:

- those in which an individual, or one member of a couple has already developed the condition;

- those in which an individual or one member of a couple is at 50% risk:
- those in which an individual or one member of a couple is at 25% risk.

The next section describes some of the issues which will be discussed with each of these groups. The discussions will vary depending on how long the family have known about Huntington's disease.

Genetic counselling for someone diagnosed with Huntington's disease

Several circumstances may result in genetic counselling being offered to someone with Huntington's disease (and their partner). An obvious time is when a diagnosis has just been made, and the family history of the disease has been either unknown or previously misunderstood. In this case you may experience a variety of emotions, but feelings of anger, anxiety, or frustration are all understandable. The counsellor may need to spend time with you going over information which you were given around the time of the diagnosis. This is because the shock you feel when you were given the diagnosis may have prevented you from understanding fully what was being said.

People frequently ask, 'Where has the disease come from?' As we saw in Chapter 4, a new diagnosis could be the result of a new mutation, but this is extremely unusual. It is more likely that the family history has been unknown because of the early death of a parent, adoption, separation of the family, or the symptoms of Huntington's disease in an elderly parent going unrecognized. This last possibility could happen if one of your parents had been diagnosed with a neurological condition which has some of the features of Huntington's disease, such as Parkinson's disease or multiple sclerosis. This raises the suspicion that the correct diagnosis should have been Huntington's disease. Even if the diagnosis in one of your parents was Huntington's disease it is possible that the genetic significance was either not properly explained, or, if it was, the family actively concealed the information so it still comes as a shock to you. During the course of establishing the family history it may become obvious that other relatives are also similarly affected. They and their immediate family may then seek genetic counselling as a consequence.

It is almost inevitable that either you, or your partner, will ask about prospects for the future and methods of treatment. (The details of available treatments and research are explained in Chapters 2, 3 and 8.) To some extent the answer will depend on your age and the stage of the illness at the time of diagnosis. Whilst it is important that questions are answered honestly, no-one can predict the future accurately. Replies often have to be of a general nature; phrases such as 'slowly progressive' are employed. Another way of describing the course of the condition is to suggest that there is unlikely to be much difference in your condition from year to year, but people who know you will notice a difference over a period of a few years.

If your family history is well known at the time of diagnosis, then discussions may turn on the way the condition was managed in the previous generation and the impact it has had on you and your family.

You may want to discuss practical issues such as driving and the ability to continue working; these have been discussed in Chapter 2.

Most people will have completed their family by the time a diagnosis of Huntington's disease is made, so their children will now be known to be at risk of developing the disorder. Genetic counsellors will not make you tell your adult children about the condition. However, assuming that the children are in the adult age range, the diagnosis of Huntington's disease has implications for their health, the future health of their children (i.e. your grandchildren), and for decisions they may be making about having or extending their own family. If you ask the question: 'Should we tell the children about Huntington's disease?' then a genetic counsellor may not answer directly, but reply along the lines of 'What are your concerns about talking to the children about Huntington's disease?'

Most parents worry about whether, and how, to tell children. They can benefit from a discussion of the general issues involved and the specific concerns for their family. Telling your children gives them options including: doing nothing, seeking information in their own right, deciding for themselves whether to start or extend their family, having a predictive test, or considering a prenatal test. These options are explained in more detail in the next section. While it is understandable to feel that by not informing the children you are protecting them (particularly as there is no treatment to prevent Huntington's disease) this is frequently not really the case. It is unlikely that you can conceal the diagnosis and genetic implications in the long term as there is much more publicity about

Huntington's disease in the media and in schools than there has been in the past. If your children do find out about Huntington's disease some other way they will probably feel angry on the grounds that they should have been given the opportunity to make their own informed choices. Whilst finding out about Huntington's disease can never be good news, it is my own experience that people do not like being kept in the dark about important issues which directly affect them.

If your children are young, then time is available to consider the best method of informing them. Parents sometimes feel they must wait until the 'right time', but this can mean that it is very difficult to decide when is the 'right' time. Putting off a discussion until school examinations are over, or until the child has grown up and is in a steady relationship, has the disadvantage that the information can come as a shock. Another disadvantage is that the child may well guess some of the implications, but, sensing a family secret, has felt unable to discuss them with you. Whilst it is not possible to be dogmatic about the 'right' age to tell children, many parents feel it is best to start feeding them some information at an early age. It is possible to encourage children to ask questions and then to give answers which are appropriate for their age and understanding. Over time, children grow up with the knowledge that one of their parents has Huntington's disease and the implications for themselves. It comes as less of a shock, family relationships are easier to maintain, and in due course the children are able to make their own decisions about how to deal with their risk.

An essential component of the genetic counselling process is to offer support. You need to feel that you can re-contact the clinic as and when necessary. In this context, you need to know that further help and information is available when either you or your children request it. The counsellor may give you the address of the patients' organization. No-one is forced to join, but you have the option of making contact if and when you are ready. The patients' organization has leaflets and booklets which, among others, can help you come to terms with your own diagnosis, caring for a relative with Huntington's disease, or telling your children about the condition.

Similar considerations apply to telling your brothers and sisters and other relatives about the diagnosis. Occasionally, difficulties with relationships in a family mean that giving information takes time. It is better for genetic counsellors to work with families rather than force issues and impose genetic counselling on them as this is likely to be counterproductive. Genetic counsellors are frequently able to maintain contact with some members of either your close or extended family, so in most cases, and over time, they can be sure that relevant members of your extended family are aware of the diagnosis of Huntington's disease. In this way your other relatives are able to choose whether and when to seek further help and information.

Genetic counselling for an individual at 50% risk

This is a common reason for referral. You may have known about the risks of Huntington's disease in the family for some time and now feel you want more information about the genetic aspects. This can be for a variety of reasons: you may want to discuss genetic tests, you may have plans for marriage or starting a family, or you may want to talk to your children and need to know about yourself first. Alternatively, you may have discovered the risks of Huntington's disease following a new diagnosis in your parent and need information. In either case, you may attend the clinic alone, or, if appropriate, attend as a couple in which one partner has an affected parent. The nature of the discussion will vary depending on the particular circumstances, but there are specific areas which are usually covered as described below.

Risk estimation

As Huntington's disease is inherited in an autosomal dominant manner (see Chapter 4 for further details), anyone with an affected parent has a 50% chance of inheriting the disease. As we saw in Chapter 1, the disease often starts between the ages of 35 years and 55 years, so as you become older and remain well it is less likely that you have inherited the gene.

One way to think about this is to consider 200 people born on the same day with an affected parent, as shown in Figure 18. On average, 100 of them will have the gene and 100 will not. The chance of anyone in that group having the gene is 100/200 = 50%. It is known that Huntington's disease can develop at almost any age but if we accept that half the people with the gene develop the condition before the age of 45 years then we can consider what will have happened when the group

(a)

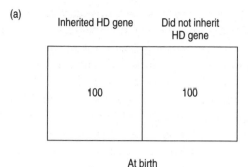

(b)

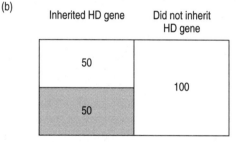

Figure 18. Diagram to show the risk of 200 people with an affected parent born on the same day. In (a), if we think about this then 100 people will have the gene and 100 will not, but we cannot tell which is which so the risk is 100/200 = 50%. As we saw from Chapter 1, half the people with the gene will show signs of Huntington's disease before the age of 45 years. Therefore, in (b) 50 will be affected, 50 people will have the gene but not yet have a problem, and 100 never had the gene. The risk that a healthy individual has the gene is now 50/150 = 33%.

of 200 people reach the age of 45 years. By this age, 50 of them will have shown signs of the disease, 50 of them will have the gene but not yet be affected and

100 of them will not have inherited the gene. There are now only 150 people in the group who have no features of Huntington's disease; therefore, the chance that one of these individuals has the gene is 50/150 = 33%. The chance that a healthy individual has not inherited the gene is 100/150 = 66%. The risk estimate is not based on the chance of you inheriting the gene, but on the chance of you developing Huntington's disease *after* the age at which you came to the clinic. Similar calculations can be done for any age and the results plotted on a curve (Figure 19). This curve is based on the age of onset figures from a survey in South Wales. There have been other surveys that give slightly different figures, but the general principles are the same. The basic point is that the

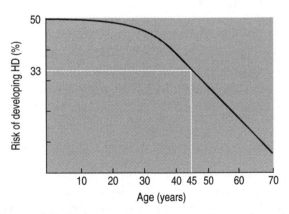

Figure 19. Risk curve for someone with an affected parent. As the person gets older *and* remains healthy the chance of developing Huntington's disease in the future gets less. Someone who is still healthy at 45 years has a 33% chance of developing the condition in the future. The risks do not fall appreciably until after middle age.

risk of developing Huntington's disease does not significantly decline until after the age when most people consider having children. We can now distinguish two types of risk; the *prior risk*, which is the chance of inheriting the gene; and the *modified risk*, which is based on age. In this section we are mainly concerned with people who have a prior risk of 50%. If you have a prior risk of 50% you may have children; these children have a prior risk of 25% because they have an affected grandparent. This is adjusted to half your modified risk, so in the case of a 45-year-old with an age-modified risk of 33%, the chance of his or her children developing Huntington's disease is 16–17%. Both these risks will become smaller as the 45-year-old person gets older and stays well.

People with a prior risk of 50% sometimes ask if their children can develop Huntington's disease before them. Although some very exceptional cases have been described in the medical literature where this may have happened, it is possible to be reassuring on this point: the vast majority of children do not develop features of Huntington's disease ahead of a parent at 50% risk.

Telling the children about Huntington's disease

Many people who discover that they have a 50% prior risk will have young children. If this is the case you and your partner have to decide whether to tell the children about Huntington's disease being in the family, and if so when and how. The general issues and principles involved have been discussed in the previous section. Some people decide to talk openly about the family history so that their children are used to hearing about Huntington's disease from an early age. Many people have told me about their experiences of discussing the implications of Huntington's disease with their children and I have been struck by the acceptance and resilience of young people.

There are some additional points about telling children if you are at 50% risk. Clearly, you have to have some acceptance of your own risk first. Another dilemma is whether to worry your children because it may not be necessary if you are not a gene carrier. Not telling them seems attractive at first sight, but the shock is all the greater if you develop Huntington's disease or are found to be a gene carrier when tested.

Options discussed by genetic counsellors before the gene was identified

An important issue for those at 50% risk is the implications for having a family. Before the mid 1980s the choices were:

● not to have children at all, or not to extend your family (depending on the timing of receiving information about Huntington's disease)
● in the case of a male at risk for Huntington's disease there was (and remains) the possibility for the partner to have children by artificial insemination by a donor
● to have children and accept the risk

All three options have their drawbacks. For some couples the option of not having children was acceptable despite the obvious drawback of possibly discovering later in life that they were unaffected. Although some couples finding out about Huntington's disease in middle age say: 'If we had known about Huntington's disease earlier we would not have had children', the desire to have children is strong. Many younger couples felt the right decision for them was to have children and accept the risk. In the case of males at risk for Huntington's disease, having children using donor sperm gets around the genetic problem; however, it was not an option chosen by many couples. The localization of the gene in 1983 and subsequent identification 10 years later in 1993 (see Chapter 4 for details) means that additional options are now available, including:

- predictive testing
- prenatal diagnosis
- exclusion testing in pregnancy
- depositing DNA for possible future use

These additional options started to become available from the mid 1980s, but were limited to a few couples because the genetic tests during that period relied heavily on family studies and the appropriate family structure was frequently unavailable. The identification of the gene in 1993 simplified the laboratory aspects of the tests. However, while no effective treatment is available, the genetic counselling aspects described in the next section remain. The genetic counselling and laboratory tests are available in most countries of Western Europe, North America, and Australasia. In Britain predictive testing is organized as part of the National Health Service so you do not have to pay for the test. It is beyond the scope of this book to give details of methods of paying for health care in other countries.

Genetic counselling for predictive testing

Predictive testing is a method of determining whether an individual has inherited the Huntington's disease gene *before* the onset of the disease. Several different types of predictive test were considered in the past, but there were doubts about their reliability and so they were never used. The new test currently available examines the genetic material directly and is therefore much more reliable. The recommended approach to predictive testing is written in international guidelines. Before describing what is involved in a predictive test we need to consider why these guidelines were established.

Need for guidelines for predictive testing

When predictive testing became a real possibility, there was concern that people might have their blood tested without first having genetic counselling. There was also a worry about the potential misuse of the information by others in society. The basic problem is that a positive result indicates that a gene carrier will develop a progressive neurological illness, at some time in the future, for which no effective treatment is available. Therefore, there is no direct advantage, in medical terms, in knowing that you carry the gene. In addition, there were fears that people would take the test without thinking through the implications and regretting the decision afterwards.

An international committee, composed of members of the World Federation of Neurology Research Group on Huntington's disease and members from the International Huntington's Association, which is the patients' organization, prepared the guidelines. These guidelines do not have the force of law, but establish a framework for doctors from different countries to provide predictive tests in a consistent way. Guidelines cannot cover every situation, but they do help to set out the basic principles. In addition, they form the basis for further discussion and, unlike laws, can be modified easily in the light of experience or new information. The description of the predictive test which follows is based on those guidelines.

Counselling aspects

The guidelines clearly state that anyone requesting a predictive test needs a minimum of two counselling sessions, separated by at least one month, before receiving a test result at a third session. In practice, there may be more than a month between the two sessions. At first glance this seems dictatorial, and it is therefore important for you to understand why this is recommended, and to know some of the areas which will be discussed.

You (and your partner) and the counsellor need the chance to think through the consequences of a positive test result as well as the consequences of a negative result. Each counsellor is different, but you will probably be asked why you think the test is in your best interest. There may be a mixture of reasons why you are considering a predictive test, but people often say that they need to know for themselves: that is, certainty is better than uncertainty. This is without doubt the most common reason given to me. You may also want definite information so that you know what to say to your children or to help you decide about starting a family. You will also be asked how you and your family will feel if the test shows you have the gene and how you will feel if the test shows you do not have the gene. In fact, neither you nor anyone else can say exactly how you will react to being told that you will develop Huntington's disease in the future, or, conversely, that you are no longer at risk. The counsellor can tell you how other couples have reacted and can tell you the results of studies of predictive testing which have been reported in the medical literature. However, the counsellor cannot say how *you* will react. In general, the number of adverse effects of having a positive test, in terms of serious depression or suicide have been few. It is possible that these severe reactions were due to onset of the disease coinciding with the test result. It is natural for anyone receiving bad news to feel upset or down for a time, but most individuals or couples recover over a relatively short period. If you are in a stable relationship then a reason to have your partner present during the predictive testing sessions is to provide support for you. However, it may be the case that your partner is more upset than you are if the result indicates that you are going to develop Huntington's disease, as your partner also has to come to terms with a sense of loss.

You might expect that a negative result is good news for you. Indeed it is, but some people have felt guilty that they have escaped whereas other members of their family have not. Some people have felt a little frustrated because they spent years worrying needlessly about Huntington's disease. After the relief of knowing that you have not got the gene you will have to come back to the reality of dealing with common worries such as jobs, money, or relationships.

Other areas for discussion could include possible effects on any children, as a positive result will mean that their prior risks are automatically elevated from 25% to 50%. Depending on the circumstances, it may be appropriate to discuss the possibility of pre-natal tests. Similarly it may be relevant for an individual or couple to consider the effect of a positive predictive test result on any future insurance proposal or other legal contract. For young adults, in particular, implications for further education, training, and employment may need to be considered as well.

Special circumstances may arise if the counsellor is worried that you are already showing signs of depression. If this happens then there may be a need to consider postponing the test until a psychiatrist has had an opportunity to ensure that treatment for depression and additional support are available. Another area of difficulty is when the counsellor detects the early clinical signs of the disease, but the person seeking the test is seemingly unaware of them. If the counsellor is confident about the clinical signs then it is inevitable that the test will be positive. One way of dealing with this is to ask if the individual or partner is worried that Huntington's disease has already started. Another way is to ask if the person would like to be examined *and* know the results of a clinical neurological examination, after which any suspicions can be discussed.

Some centres may offer the predictive test on a purely service basis, whilst others may be collecting information in a systematic way as part of a research project. If there is a research project being conducted in addition to the test then your participation in the research will be voluntary.

Your counsellor will spend time describing the technical aspects of the test. Many centres ask for a written consent form to be signed before the blood is taken for the test. This form confirms the major points which were discussed and your agreement to being tested. The counsellor will also need to discuss the manner in which the result will be delivered. The guidelines are specific: this should be done in person and not via the telephone or by letter. The guidelines also lay down that testing centres should have the ability to provide counselling and support after the test result. The counsellor will also explain the arrangements for professional support when you receive the result. You will also want to think about which relatives and friends you will tell as part of your own support system. Some people have also chosen to discuss the results with their employers whilst others would never consider this. Testing centres are very concerned that confidentiality should be the rule. The results of a predictive test should not be disclosed to anyone else without your permission, but it is customary for your family doctor to be informed. This has the obvious advantage that they can be part of the support mechanism. Very occasionally, I have had requests that the family doctor should not be informed and have agreed to this after the reasons have been explained.

Given the need to have a wide-ranging discussion and to impart technical information it is not surprising that more than one session is required.

Although some people complain that this prolongs the testing procedure, it has the advantage that you have been able to discuss all the issues involved, some of which you may not have previously considered. You have the opportunity to think about both the advantages and disadvantages of the test, and this will help you to make an informed final decision. Taking two sessions also means that your decision has been consistent over a period of time. This is especially important for those who have only recently learnt that they are at risk because of a new diagnosis in the family. A decision to go ahead with the test when you may be shocked or angry needs to be considered carefully. If more sessions are needed then these will be arranged.

The majority of people will have their predictive test according to the guidelines, but the guidelines can be modified in exceptional circumstances, such as someone coming to the clinic when they are already several weeks pregnant. Providing genetic counselling when a pregnancy is underway is always less than ideal because decisions about tests have to be taken quickly if they are to influence whether or not to continue the pregnancy.

Finally, the age at which someone can have a predictive test needs to be considered. The guidelines state that the person should have reached the age of majority for the relevant country. In the UK that is 18 years, although consent after 16 years is usually acceptable. The intention behind the guideline is that the person should be mature. Unfortunately, there is nothing magic about 18, or any other age for that matter; one individual could be very mature at 16 and another very immature at 19 or 20. In any event there is no intention to test young children.

Technical aspects of the test

As part of the process of ensuring informed choice, you need to understand some of the technical aspects of the laboratory test. It may be easiest to begin with the basics and remind you that we have two copies of our genes and that they are packaged on to chromosomes (see Chapter 4 for further details). The gene for Huntington's disease is on chromosome 4. Your affected parent has one normal copy of the gene and one which causes Huntington's disease. The copy of the gene which causes Huntington's disease has a part which is larger than normal. You are bound to have a normal-sized copy of the gene from your unaffected parent. The question is, did you inherit the normal-sized copy from your affected parent, in which case Huntington's disease will not develop, or, alternatively, did you inherit the larger copy, in which case you will develop Huntington's disease at some time in the future. The chance of the result being positive, that is that Huntington's disease has been inherited, is based on your age-modified risk, which has already been described. If you are in your twenties this is still effectively 50% but if you are aged 45 years it is 33%, and if you are older it will be even lower.

If you decide to go ahead, then your genetic material will be extracted from a sample of blood and it is a relatively easy laboratory procedure to assess the sizes of the genes. There is a small overlap between the normal size and the Huntington's disease size (see Fig. 14, p. 53) so three types of result are possible:

- clearly in the normal range (negative)
- in the grey area around normal size and Huntington's disease size, in which case it may be difficult to interpret the result (see Fig. 14)

- clearly in the Huntington's disease size range (positive)

The grey area is small, so, in the majority of cases, the results are clearly normal (negative) or clearly abnormal (positive). Although no medical test can be described as 100% accurate, the chances of error involved in direct tests of the gene are extremely small, but difficult to calculate. The test can be described as **close to** 100% accurate. It is my practice to ask the laboratory to process two samples of blood separately in the hope that this will prevent people worrying at a later date 'Did they get it right?'. As a further precaution, the testing centre may check that a positive test result has been obtained on an affected member of your family. Checking that an affected relative has a positive result does remove the, admittedly remote, possibility that Huntington's disease is not the correct diagnosis in the family.

The test itself can be done in a few days, if necessary, but practical considerations, either within the laboratory or for yourselves, mean that it usually takes a little longer—but it should be weeks rather than months before the result is known.

As we saw on p. 53 the size of the gene is unhelpful in predicting the age of onset for any particular person. In order to prevent confusion, some centres will not tell you the exact size of the gene, but just give the result as positive or negative. This is undoubtedly true for results over 40 repeats. On p. 57 I explained that in exceptional cases someone with a repeat size in the range of 36–39 repeats could develop Huntington's disease at the usual time, or very late in life, or even have died before the condition starts. If the result of a predictive test is in this range then a genetic counsellor may have to explain this possibility to you, but also emphasize that your children would still be at risk of developing Huntington's disease.

Are there problems with results just under 36 repeats?

Very occasionally someone will have a result of say 33 repeats. This could just as easily come from the unaffected side of the family. On p. 56 I mentioned that new mutations can occur, and this result is in the range which may give rise to a new mutation in a future generation. The interpretation of this type of result is difficult. It is less than 36 repeats so you will not develop Huntington's disease. However, the counsellor will have to let you know that there is still a small risk for your children and grandchildren. Fortunately, results in the range which can give rise to new mutations do not occur very often.

Do predictive tests affect insurance?

A fundamental principle of an insurance policy is that you and the company act in good faith. This means that you have to declare all relevant information to the company at the time you take out the policy. If you took out a policy, and answered all the questions honestly, before finding out about Huntington's disease or before having a predictive test then you need have no concern.

Scientists and doctors involved in providing predictive tests for Huntington's disease, and other disorders, were concerned that anyone who has a positive result would be unable to obtain any insurance *in the future*. A worse concern was that insurance companies could coerce people into having predictive tests when they applied for a new policy. The insurance industry sells many different types of policies, but the main focus of concern is with those policies which are linked to house purchase and health care. In a country, such as the UK, which has an effective National Health Service funded by general taxes this is less of an issue. Of course, the position varies from country to country. Many people in the UK use insurance policies to help pay the mortgage on their homes. The insurance industry in the UK has established a voluntary code which means that:

- They will not ask anyone to have a genetic test.
- Whilst they may take the family history into account, if you have a positive test and apply for life insurance linked to a mortgage of under £100 000 then the companies will ignore the results.
- This response from the insurance industry in the UK is initially for a short period but in all likelihood it will become standard practice for the future.

Other countries have different social structures and have taken alternative approaches to this problem. In my experience, insurance is not a major issue for most people who come for predictive testing.

Prenatal testing

Prenatal diagnosis is a method of detecting, in the early stages of pregnancy, whether a fetus has, or has not, inherited the Huntington's disease gene. As with predictive testing, the issues involved have to be considered carefully. If you know you have inherited the gene as a result of a predictive test (or possibly because of the onset of the condition) you might want to think about prenatal diagnosis. If cells of fetal origin are obtained early in the course of a pregnancy then the same laboratory techniques as were described previously may be used to determine whether the fetus has inherited the Huntington's disease gene. If the result is negative then the decision to continue the pregnancy is straightforward. Alternatively, if the result is positive then you have to consider termination of pregnancy. Termination of a wanted pregnancy is obviously very traumatic and needs to be discussed sensitively. An important point to realize is that if the result is positive and you then refuse a termination, the child will be born with the certainty of developing Huntington's disease in the future. If this happens, then the child will grow up with the knowledge that he or she is going to develop Huntington's disease and will have been denied the opportunity to decide whether to have the test as an adult. Ideally, the counsellor will discuss these issues well before a pregnancy so that you are able to come to terms with the possible outcomes of a prenatal test.

Apart from the genetic aspects of prenatal diagnosis, the obstetric aspects must also be considered; these are essentially the same whatever the genetic condition. There are two common methods of obtaining fetal cells; the first is called **chorion biopsy** (variations on the name include chorion villus sampling or CVS); and the second is called **amniocentesis**. Each of these obstetric procedures has advantages and disadvantages.

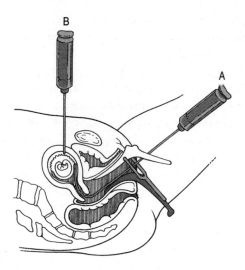

Figure 20. The technique of chorion biopsy. In this procedure the obstetrician wants to obtain cells from
the placenta or afterbirth. There are two ways of
approaching the placenta. One way is through the neck
of the womb and the other is through the skin of the
abdomen. Both approaches are shown on the diagram
but of course only one would be chosen. In either case
an ultrasound machine is used to help guide the
obstetrician.

Chorion biopsy involves taking a small piece of
the placenta or afterbirth at about 10–11 weeks into
the pregnancy as shown in Figure 20. There are two
ways of reaching the placenta; one is to pass a
catheter through the vagina and neck of the womb;
the other method involves passing a needle through
the skin of the abdomen. Whichever method is
chosen, an ultrasound scan guides the obstetrician
to the correct place. It is very important to realize
that the needle or catheter is not put into the fetus.

The biopsy will contain both fetal and maternal tissue; the maternal tissue can be stripped away in the laboratory, leaving enough fetal tissue for the DNA test. The result should be available before the twelfth week of the pregnancy. If you require a termination this can be undertaken using a general anaesthetic. The main disadvantage of the chorion biopsy procedure is the risk of miscarriage. Each antenatal clinic quotes slightly different risk figures, but approximately 2% (2 in 100) is reasonable. The procedure can also be done later in the pregnancy, but most couples find it possible to contact an appropriate centre soon after a pregnancy has been confirmed. The advantages of obtaining results in the first three months of pregnancy include: having a test when knowledge of the pregnancy can still be private to the couple concerned, and if there is a need to have a termination it can be performed by a less distressing method.

The alternative procedure, amniocentesis, involves taking some fluid from around the 'baby' at approximately 16 weeks. This fluid contains some fetal cells which can be grown in culture and used in the DNA test. Although the risk of miscarriage is said to be 1/2–1% (compared with 2% for chorion biopsy), the test result is available later in the pregnancy. If you require a termination this would be done by inducing a miscarriage which is likely to be more distressing. For this reason the majority of couples opt for the earlier test.

Storing DNA

After discussion, you may come to the conclusion that you do not want a predictive test, but would rather leave a sample of DNA in storage at the testing centre so that it is available for analysis after death for the benefit of your children. It would also be available for analysis in the future if you change your mind about a predictive test. When your children are adults they can have a test in their own right. However, if you were to die early it would be easier to test your sample, since if it is negative your children do not need any further tests. If it is positive then each child can decide whether or not to have tests for themselves.

Genetic counselling for exclusion testing in pregnancy

The description of the discovery of the Huntington's disease gene is given in Chapter 4. An essential step was the discovery, in 1983, that the gene for Huntington's disease is on chromosome 4, although its precise position was not known until 1993. There were a series of markers, or variations in the DNA, close to the gene, which could be traced through a family in order to provide genetic information to those at risk. Essentially, these markers are present in every family and by themselves are not useful. However, in a family with Huntington's disease, if a specific marker was shown to be inherited with the gene, then predictive information was obtained for those at risk. The main problem with this type of test was that it required a family study of at least two living, and ideally three, generations. In practice most Huntington's disease families were too small to make use of the technology. One application was, and remains, the exclusion test in pregnancy. In this analysis the three generations are made up from a

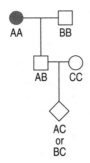

Figure 21. Diagram to illustrate an exclusion test in pregnancy. The markers A, B, and C represent natural variations in the DNA molecule close to the Huntington's disease gene. The way of working out whether the risk to the fetus has increased or decreased is given in the text.

couple with partner at 50% risk, the parent of the person at risk, and the fetus, as shown in Figure 21. In the example, the person at risk inherited marker A from his affected parent and marker B from his unaffected parent. By itself this gives no extra information, except to say that marker A is associated with the risk of Huntington's disease and marker B is not. If the fetus inherits marker B then it has inherited the chromosome 4 from its unaffected grandparent; therefore, Huntington's disease has been excluded. Conversely, if the fetus inherits marker A the risk has increased from 25% to 50%. Huntington's disease has not been excluded, but equally it is not definite that the fetus will develop Huntington's disease. The parents risk has not altered; the only question being asked in this test is: 'Did the fetus inherit the chromosome 4 which came from its affected grandparent or did it inherit the chromosome 4 from its unaffected grandparent?' As this is an indirect method of studying the gene there is a small error associated with the test that is of the order of 1–2%. Another point to realize is that if Huntington's disease is not excluded, the at-risk parent and the fetus have inherited the same chromosome 4 from the affected grandparent and now have the same genetic risks (barring the small error because the test is indirect).

If the fetus has inherited the chromosome 4 from its affected grandparent and is now at 50% risk, then you have a difficult decision regarding terminating the pregnancy. Both you and the fetus share the same chromosome as the affected grandparent. If you continue the pregnancy and at some point in the future you develop Huntington's disease, it will be clear that your child is also going to be affected. Your child will then grow up knowing that he or she is definitely going to develop Huntington's disease, rather than just being at risk. The child will have had no opportunity to make an individual decision about whether to be tested as an adult. On the other hand, if you terminate the pregnancy and do not develop Huntington's disease in the future then you will know that your offspring would not have developed it either. If you do decide that exclusion testing is a good option for you, the genetic counsellor will help you come to terms with these choices prior to a pregnancy.

The description of the obstetric procedures involved is the same as that given in the section on prenatal diagnosis.

Since the identification of the gene, this type of test is less relevant to most couples at risk for Huntington's disease. However, it is occasionally considered when someone does not want a predictive test, but does want children free from risk, and artificial insemination by donor is unacceptable or inappropriate. It has to be said that this test is complex and still provokes controversy among doctors because, on average, half of all pregnancies tested in this way will be terminated on the basis of a 50% risk which means that, on average, half the fetuses terminated will not have inherited the gene.

Genetic counselling for an individual at 25% risk

The identification of the gene means that genetic tests no longer require complex family studies. It is now technically possible for anyone with an affected grandparent but with an unaffected parent (who has not had, or does not want a predictive test) to be tested. However, if you are in this position, in addition to the general points about predictive testing, the counsellor will want to discuss the effects of the result on the rest of the family. Clearly, if you are shown to have the gene, then your unaffected parent must also have the gene and your brothers and sisters will be at 50% risk. On the other hand, if you do not have the gene, then other family members cannot infer any information about themselves. This is because it is still possible for the gene to be present in your at-risk parent, even though your parent is currently unaffected. Unless there has been complete fragmentation of the family, it is unlikely that you could keep a positive result completely secret. The counsellor will ask whether it is possible for you to tell your at-risk parent what you are planning before the test is carried out. It is obviously up to you whether you have the test, but your counsellor will want to know you have thought through the impact of the test on your particular family.

Pre-implantation genetic testing

This is an idea which makes use of the techniques of *in vitro* fertilization (IVF) and doing genetic tests on embryos. It has an advantage over prenatal exclusion testing in that a termination of pregnancy is not required, but instead involves all the emotional issues surrounding IVF. This is still at an early stage of development so further details cannot be given in this chapter.

Conclusion

Genetic counselling is a process which allows you to obtain accurate information about Huntington's disease. The counsellor wants to help you come to terms with the fact that Huntington's disease has occurred in your family and give you time to choose your best option given your particular circumstances. Although much has been made of recent developments in predictive testing, only about 15–20% of people at risk for Huntington's disease choose this option.

The localization of the Huntington's disease to chromosome 4 and its subsequent identification has increased the range of options available for people at risk for Huntington's disease. The initial fears that predictive testing would have major adverse effects precipitated a dialogue between professionals interested in Huntington's disease and the patients' organizations which resulted in the development of guidelines. Although individuals select themselves for predictive testing, there have been few serious adverse effects. This may, in part, be due to the careful genetic counselling accompanying the test.

It needs to be emphasized that identifying the gene for Huntington's disease was not an end in itself, nor was its purpose solely to develop predictive tests or tests in pregnancy. The objective was, and remains, to increase the basic understanding of Huntington's disease in the hope that this will lead to more effective treatment.

6
Changes in the brain

As you might expect, the changes which occur in the brain of someone with Huntington's disease have been studied in great detail over many years. In this chapter I want to describe this pattern of change. It is interesting in itself but also helps to understand some of the ideas for further research which will be described in the next two chapters.

What is a nerve cell?

The brain contains millions of nerve cells. Figure 22 shows a diagram of a typical nerve cell. It consists of a main area called the **nerve cell body**, which is covered in **projections**. Most of the projections are small and these receive impulses from other nerve cells. There is one larger projection, called an **axon**, which is covered in fatty material. This axon transmits impulses to another part of the nervous system. A nerve cell receives an impulse because a chemical is transmitted from the end of one nerve cell to one

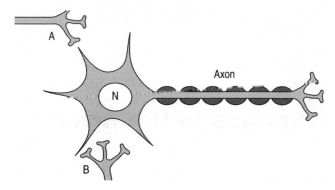

Figure 22. The parts of a nerve cell. The genetic material is found in the nucleus of the cell, N. The main part of the nerve cell is covered in projections so that it can receive chemical messages from other nerve cells (represented by A and B in this diagram). The nerve cell has a long projection called the 'axon' which may or may not be covered by fatty material. The nerve can transmit signals to another part of the nervous system via chemical messages from the end of the axon.

of the projections on the other cell. If the nerve cell bodies are collected together in an area of the brain it will have a grey colour, whereas areas of the brain which contain the long projections covered in fatty material appear white.

Are there any changes to be seen on just looking at the brain?

One of the first things a doctor will notice when looking at the brain of someone who has died after many years of Huntington's disease is that the brain is slightly smaller, weighs a little less, and the folds on the surface are a little wider than the brain of

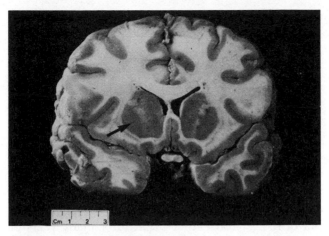

Figure 23. Photograph of a cut brain from a normal individual. The surface of the brain is the cortex and is grey. The fatty material on the axons makes part of the brain appear white. There is another large area of grey in the middle of the picture (*arrowed*) which is the basal ganglia. (Reproduced with the permission of W.B. Saunders.)

someone the same age who died of something completely different, say a heart attack. This change could occur in a lot of neurological disorders, and further work needs to be done to recognize the pattern of changes typical of Huntington's disease.

Are there changes to be seen when the brain is cut?

If the brain is cut, the pattern of damage becomes apparent. If you look at the picture of the normal brain in Figure 23 you can see that there is grey matter around the outside and white matter in the middle. The grey matter around the outside of the brain is called the **cortex**. At the base of the brain more grey matter can be seen. This area of grey matter contains more nerve cells and is called the **basal ganglia**. In this section of the brain, the grey matter is in two parts which are called the **caudate nucleus** and the **putamen**. The shape of the basal ganglia is important. The caudate nucleus bulges into what appears to be a space. (In life this space is filled with fluid.)

If you now look at a similar section of someone who died of Huntington's disease (Figure 24) you can see that the folds on the surface are wider, but, more importantly, the basal ganglia are reduced to a rim of tissue. You can see that after many years of Huntington's disease there is considerable damage to the basal ganglia. In fact, similar changes can be seen on a brain scan during life.

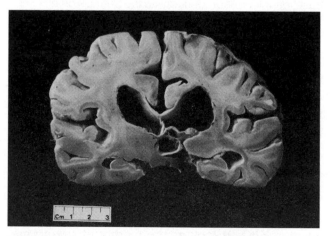

Figure 24. Photograph of the cut surface of the brain of someone with Huntington's disease. It is clear that there has been considerable damage to the basal ganglia. (Reproduced with the permission of W.B. Saunders.)

As we saw in Chapter 4, we now have a very reliable genetic test. Before the genetic test was available, pathologists were asked to examine the brains of people who had died of an illness which could have been Huntington's disease. The question arose as to whether the pathologist could give an absolutely definite diagnosis. The answer to this was 'not quite'. The pathologist acts in much the same way as other doctors when making a diagnosis: they try to recognize particular patterns. If there were doubts about a diagnosis when someone was alive then it was very helpful if a pathologist reported that the pattern of change in the brain was typical of Huntington's disease.

Are other areas of the brain affected?

The answer to this is 'yes'. Although the brunt of the damage occurs to the basal ganglia, subtle changes occur to other areas of the brain. These can be seen with the help of a microscope, but need not be considered in detail in this book: instead, I want to say more about the basal ganglia.

What is the function of the basal ganglia?

If the basal ganglia are badly damaged in Huntington's disease, then it is very reasonable to ask what functions do the basal ganglia normally control and how does the damage relate to the clinical features which were described in Chapters 2 and 3? At a very simple level we could suggest that the nerve cells in the basal ganglia are involved in co-ordinating activity in the cortex to signal changes in various muscles to give a smooth pattern of movements. A similar co-ordinating role probably applies to give a smooth sequence of thoughts. The next question is 'How'?

Although this is far from clear, we have an understanding of a series of connections between the cortex and the basal ganglia involved in co-ordinating movement. Figure 25(a) and (b) shows a simplified diagram of some of these connections. There are two pathways from the caudate and putamen nuclei: a longer route which is called the **indirect pathway** and a shorter one called the **direct pathway**. As nerve cells in the caudate and putamen are lost, both these pathways are damaged in Huntington's disease.

The output of a nerve cell can either **excite** or **inhibit** the next nerve cell in the pathway. If a nerve cell is excited it will send more messages to the next nerve cell; conversely, if it is inhibited it will

Figure 25. Diagrams of the (a) indirect and (b) direct pathways from the basal ganglia. The basal ganglia (caudate and putamen) are damaged by Huntington's disease. The indirect pathway (a) involves loss of inhibitory impulses to the external globus pallidus (EGP). This means that there is much more inhibition of the subthalamus (STN) which means less excitation of the internal globus pallidus (IGP). This means there is less inhibition of the thalamus, which in turn means more stimulation back to the cortex. Loss of the direct pathway (b) means that there is less inhibition of the internal globus pallidus (IGP) and therefore more inhibition of the thalamus and less stimulation back to the cortex. ⊖ indicates inhibitory signals; ⊕ indicates excitatory signals.

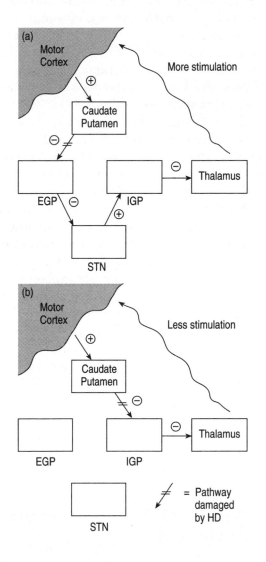

send fewer. The combination of inhibitory and excitatory signals in the pathways is confusing. The motor cortex sends excitatory signals to the caudate and putamen, but as these cells are damaged the balance of the indirect and direct pathways is altered. This is the key point, but we can consider the pathways in more detail.

The indirect pathway is shown in Figure 25(a). A decrease in inhibitory signals from the caudate and putamen allows the *external globus pallidus* to send more inhibitory signals to the *subthalamus*. The output of the subthalamus is excitatory but as it is now more inhibited this leads to less excitation of the *internal globus pallidus*. The output of the internal globus pallidus is inhibitory so fewer inhibitory signals are sent to the thalamus. Overactivity of the thalamus back to the cortex probably explains the chorea.

Damage to the direct pathway in Figure 25(b) leads to more inhibition of the thalamus. More inhibition of the thalamus reduces stimulation of the cortex and probably explains the slow movements which are seen in Huntington's disease. Relatively speaking, the indirect pathway is damaged earlier in the course of the disease, which explains why chorea is a prominent sign at the start of the condition. As more nerve cells in the basal ganglia are lost so more abnormalities of movement become apparent.

Are particular cells in the caudate and putamen lost?

The answer is 'yes'. The caudate and putamen contain a mixture of cells. They can be identified by

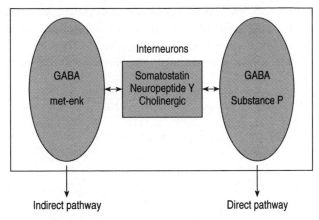

Figure 26. Diagram showing some of the different nerve cell types in the basal ganglia. Those nerve cells which contain GABA and met-enkephalin (met-enk) or GABA and substance P are particularly susceptible to loss in Huntington's disease. The interneurons which contain other neurotransmitters are relatively spared.

the chemicals which they transmit to the next nerve cell in the pathway. It is these chemicals which determine whether the effect on the next nerve cell is going to be inhibitory or stimulatory. Figure 26 shows a diagram of the cells in the caudate and putamen. In 1973 Tom Perry discovered that nerve cells which contain the chemical transmitter GABA (GABA stands for 'γ aminobutyric acid', but this long term is seldom used) are lost in Huntington's disease. We now know that a nerve cell can have more than one chemical transmitter. To make the story more complicated, there are two types of GABA cell. Some cells contain the second chemical transmitter 'met-enkephalin' and these send their chemical messages via the indirect pathway. A second group of nerve cells contain the second transmitter 'substance P' and these send their chemical messages via the direct pathway.

Some clear summary points may be made from this description:

- the loss of nerve cells in Huntington's disease is *selective*;
- cells which contain GABA are particularly sensitive to the damage caused by Huntington's disease;
- there is some explanation for the movement disorder seen in Huntington's disease;
- how the damage leads to abnormal thought processes is not clearly understood.

Having discovered which cells are particularly damaged in Huntington's disease the next questions are how and why these cells? The answer to these questions is not known, but I want to consider ways in which these questions have been addressed in the next chapter.

Can the changes in the brain explain some of the personality changes?

For many years doctors considered the basal ganglia to be mainly involved in controlling movement. The question of understanding some of the personality changes has been difficult because of confounding issues, such as depression, and the fact that the cortex is affected to some extent as well as the basal ganglia. Broadly speaking, doctors have classified dementia as either **cortical** or **sub-cortical**. Alz-

heimer's disease falls into the cortical dementia cat-
egory, because this is where most of the damage
occurs. Huntington's disease, Parkinson's disease,
and a few other rare disorders are considered to be
sub-cortical dementias. This terminology clearly
describes the fact that the basal ganglia are below
the cortex. In Huntington's disease and Parkinson's
disease the brunt of the damage is in these areas. As
a generalization, people with sub-cortical dementia
have slowed thinking and learning, but, unlike
those with cortical dementia, have not lost the
ability to comprehend.

Neuropsychologists are scientists who specialize
in testing specific thinking processes. We are all
familiar with the idea of an IQ test. In fact, this is
not one test but is composed of several tests. In
addition to the IQ test there are many tests which
try to assess various different processes. A medical
doctor sometimes uses very simple tests in the clinic,
but detailed tests take some time to complete.

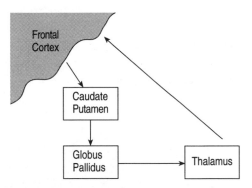

Figure 27. General diagram of the loops involved in
thought processes. The loops involve basal ganglia
(caudate and putamen) which are damaged in
Huntington's disease.

Some research programmes have been aimed at detecting differences between people with cortical dementia, or Alzheimer's disease, from those with sub-cortical dementias, such as Huntington's disease. As you might expect, different profiles are obtained in these studies. There are some similarities between people with damage to the basal ganglia and those who have just damaged the frontal part of the cortex. This is interesting as some of the planning or **executive** functions of thinking involve the front part of the brain. As with the control of motor function, so these processes involve loops of nerve cells between the frontal cortex, basal ganglia, thalamus, and back to the cortex. Figure 27 shows a general diagram of nerve loops from the frontal cortex to the basal ganglia and back again. This diagram is strikingly similar to the one on p. 101, which was used to explain the cause of the movement disorder in Huntington's disease. In Chapter 3, I described some of the personality changes which occur in Huntington's disease. Some of the difficulties which people with Huntington's disease experience: such as apathy, poor organization and planning, irritability, and inability to concentrate on several tasks, can be explained because the damage to the nerve cells in the basal ganglia upsets these nerve loops.

7
What causes selective nerve cell death?

This chapter focuses on ideas and research activity to explain why specific nerve cells die in Huntington's disease. A problem in writing this chapter is that the we do not yet have a complete explanation. This means that there are various loose ends. Understanding the detail of how the abnormal huntingtin protein results in a specific pattern of cell death is more than an academic exercise; it is essential to the development of treatments which will prevent or significantly delay the cell death in those at risk.

Are the nerve cells being murdered or do they commit suicide?

This is a dramatic way of expressing the problem. Alternatively, you could ask if the gene for Huntington's disease produces a toxic substance which kills these cells; or is there something about these cells in Huntington's disease which means that they are programmed to die back prematurely? We can consider some of the evidence for the cells being murdered by considering an animal model.

Why do we need an animal model?

An animal model allows experiments to be undertaken to answer questions about the basic problem which causes Huntington's disease. Whilst this is important, an animal model would also allow treatment options to be considered and worked out. Clearly, if a treatment slowed down the disease process in an animal model then it would be worth trying on people affected by Huntington's disease. Unfortunately, there are no animals which develop a similar disorder. This means that a similar disease has to be induced in the animal.

Are there chemicals which cause damage which is similar to Huntington's disease?

The answer to this is 'yes'. One of the chemical messengers between nerve cells is called **glutamate**. Experiments in 1969 showed that if a nerve cell receives too much excitation from glutamate then it will die. Glutamate is the chemical messenger between the cortex of the brain and the basal ganglia (Figure 25, p. 101). One model of Huntington's disease is to inject glutamate, or chemicals similar to glutamate, into the basal ganglia of a rat or a monkey and see which nerve cells are most vulnerable to the effects of the toxin. This model produces results which are surprisingly similar to the damage caused by Huntington's disease in humans. These experiments have been refined over the years so that chemicals which produce a near-perfect match with Huntington's disease have been identified.

As we saw in the last chapter, chemical messengers cross the gap between nerve cells. The chemical message is detected by receptors on the surface of the next nerve cell. Specific chemical messengers are detected by specific receptors. The experiments identified that chemicals which mimicked the damage caused by Huntington's disease used a subgroup of the glutamate receptors called NMDA. This was named after one of the chemicals which caused its stimulation.

This type of model has been very useful in helping to define which cells in the basal ganglia are especially damaged by Huntington's disease and which are relatively spared. It also suggests that the NMDA receptor is involved in the disease process. The model was developed in the 1980s before anything was known about the nature of the expansion of part of the gene or the abnormal protein, huntingtin. In this model the nerve cells are being murdered by a toxic substance.

Recent modifications to the model

Huntington's disease does not usually develop until adulthood and is slowly progressive for many years. This is completely different from injecting a toxic substance into the brain of an animal, which produces immediate damage. There are other problems with the model, including the fact that high levels of a toxic substance are not found in the brains of

people with Huntington's disease. In the early 1990s
a modification to the model was proposed.

The NMDA receptor is complex and is frequently
blocked by the nerve cell. Blocking the NMDA
receptor requires energy. Essentially, the idea is that

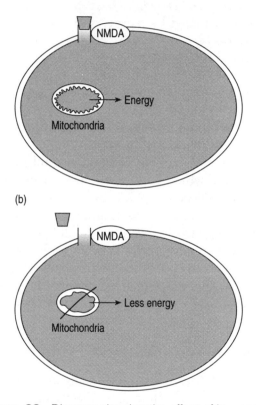

Figure 28. Diagram showing the effect of low energy
levels on the cells. In (a) the energy levels are normal
and the NMDA receptor is usually blocked. In (b) the
mitochondria are damaged so there is less energy in the
cell. The NMDA receptor is now usually open and
renders the cell susceptible to further damage.

Huntington's disease disturbs the energy levels of some cells. This in turn changes the activity of the NMDA receptor so that the cells are now susceptible to damage from normal levels of the chemical messenger (Figure 28). The energy levels of a nerve cell come from making modifications to glucose (sugar). Technically the process is called **metabolizing** glucose. Some of the metabolic process occurs in parts of the cell called **mitochondria**. Support for this theory comes from the fact that chronic injection of toxins, which damage mitochondria, into the body (not the brain) of laboratory animals can also mimic Huntington's disease. This slower damage to the brain is a better model for what happens in Huntington's disease.

Has the identification of huntingtin helped to explain the selective nerve cell loss in Huntington's disease?

In the chapter on the genetic aspects of Huntington's disease we saw that it took 10 years to move from localizing the gene to chromosome 4 to actually isolating it. It would have been marvellous if the discovery of the gene and the way in which the huntingtin protein is abnormal, had given a clue as to why some nerve cells are damaged. Unfortunately, this was not the case.

What were some of the first questions asked when huntingtin was identified?

One way of trying to determine the function of huntingtin was to see if it was similar to any other protein which had been identified. This was done and it was quickly realized that huntingtin was not similar to a protein whose function was already known.

In Chapter 4 we noted that genes are present in every cell, but in any particular cell most of the genes are inactive. The converse of this is that in any particular cell or tissue only some genes are actively making their protein product. Since some cells are selectively damaged in Huntington's disease it is reasonable to ask if huntingtin is selectively made in these cells. Again, it was soon realized that huntingtin was widely produced in all tissues, but, more importantly, was present in all nerve cells. In brain tissue from patients with Huntington's disease both the normal- and abnormal-sized proteins were made. These results were disappointing because they gave no clue to the underlying cause of the cell death in Huntington's disease. The fact that abnormal huntingtin is present in all nerve cells means that just having a longer polyglutamine tract does not, by itself, cause nerve cell death.

Another approach to the problem was to see if huntingtin was localized to a specific part of the cell. Figure 29 is a diagram showing the normal localization of huntingtin. Some of the early results were contradictory, but most studies indicated that huntingtin was not in the nucleus (which contains the

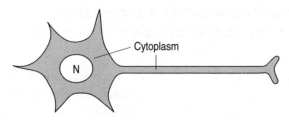

Figure 29. Diagram showing the normal position of huntingtin outside the nucleus, N.

genetic material). Normal huntingtin is found outside the nucleus, in the **cytoplasm**. Although this was progress, it still did not answer some of the basic questions about the cause of the selective cell death in Huntington's disease.

A different approach was, and still is, to identify other proteins which interact with huntingtin. Normal-sized huntingtin must interact with other proteins in the cytoplasm to produce a normal function. In the case of Huntington's disease, the larger huntingtin protein must gain a new function and this somehow leads to selective nerve cell death. Since the gene has been identified, huntingtin has been found to interact with a number of other proteins. The function of some of these proteins is known, but some of the other proteins have not been previously recognized. I have chosen not to list the various proteins with which huntingtin interacts because it is still not clear from this work how having the abnormal huntingtin leads to the selective nerve cell death typical of Huntington's disease. Naturally, there is still a lot of research work to be undertaken to characterize the interactions.

What happens if huntingtin is missing from the cell?

Another way of trying to get a handle on the function of huntingtin is to see what happens if it is missing altogether. This approach involves genetic manipulation of a mouse to damage one copy of its huntingtin gene, so that this copy does not produce any protein at all. This mouse is not remarkably different from normal; any differences which occur are subtle.

It is possible to breed mice with one copy of the gene which has been damaged and see what happens. In this type of experiment some mice ought to be born with *both* copies of the gene damaged. The interesting result was that these mice were not born, but died before birth. The conclusion from this series of experiments is that huntingtin is essential for the normal development of the brain.

The mice with one gene knocked out are not really a model of Huntington's disease because this is the complete opposite of what happens in Huntington's disease. In Huntington's disease the normal and abnormal protein are being produced. A much better animal model would be one which had a genetic modification such that the cells produce a protein with the abnormal section present.

What about the cells committing suicide?

As cells age, they die. If they died by bursting open, then the contents of the cell would damage the surrounding tissue, which would become inflamed. In order to avoid this, cells have a mechanism to quietly commit suicide without causing damage. This mechanism is sometimes called programmed cell death, and occurs in many tissues of the body. It is reasonable to ask if this mechanism is abnormal in some way in Huntington's disease and whether this is the cause of the selective nerve cell death?

Development of mice containing the first part of the human gene

It is possible to genetically modify laboratory animals, usually mice, so that a gene of interest is inserted into the genetic material. The inserted gene is called a **transgene**. It is not possible to control precisely where an inserted gene will go. However, the hope is that the gene will work and produce a protein product. A fascinating model has been the development of mice which have been genetically modified to contain the first part of the human Huntington's disease gene. Mice with this type of modification are called **transgenic**. The mice containing the first part of the gene had a very large polyglutamine expansion. In most of the mice, protein from the first part of the gene was produced. In these mice abnormal movements and neurological signs were present. These abnormal neurological signs were not entirely typical of Huntington's disease, but we have to remember that these were genetically modified mice not humans. At first, examination of the brains of the transgenic mice was disappointing: they were smaller than normal mice but otherwise not especially remarkable.

In 1997, detailed studies of the nerve cells of these mice showed that they contained clumps of protein material in the nucleus of the cell. As you will recall, this is not a part of the cell which normally contains huntingtin. These clumps of protein contained the first part of the protein. They were called **neuronal intranuclear inclusions** or **NII**. The question arose as to whether these NII were present in the nerve cells of Huntington's disease patients. Once this had been established it was soon realized that these clumps had first been seen in electron microscopic studies in 1979 but no-one had realized their significance. Since this discovery, the brains of patients with Huntington's disease have been re-examined and the NII have been found in the cortex and basal ganglia.

If you look back at the diagram of a nerve cell you will see that it has a long projection, which is called an **axon**. In 1993 it was noted that nerve cells in the cortex of Huntington's disease brains had abnormal axons. Clumps were also found in these abnormal axons.

Do the NII contain huntingtin?

In order to answer this question we have to consider the technical aspect of how huntingtin is detected in a cell. The process involves raising an **antibody** to huntingtin. We now have to consider what is an antibody. When your children were vaccinated a doctor or nurse injected proteins from a bacteria or virus into them. Your children's immune system recognized these proteins as foreign and produced antibodies specific to them. When your children encounter the live bacteria or virus their immune system immediately recognizes the foreign proteins and can now rapidly produce more relevant anti-bodies. The antibodies bind to the bacteria or virus which makes it easier for the immune system to destroy them. The vaccination programme prevents the vast majority of children from developing specific infections.

Once huntingtin was identified, antibodies were raised to the protein so that it could be detected in various parts of the cell. In these experiments the antibody is used to label the huntingtin protein. If an antibody which recognizes the central portion of huntingtin is used, then the NII are not labelled; all the huntingtin appears in the cytoplasm. However, if an antibody is used which recognizes just the very first part of huntingtin, then the NII are labelled (Figure 30). This means that huntingtin is cut and the fragments then forms clumps. How and why the fragment from abnormal huntingtin forms clumps and how and why the clumps are present in the nucleus, is unclear.

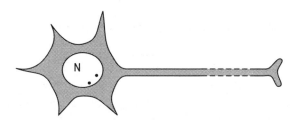

Figure 30. Diagram to show clumps inside the nucleus of cells affected by Huntington's disease. These clumps are called Neuronal Intranuclear Inclusions or NII and contain the first part of the huntingtin protein and another protein called ubiquitin. See the text for a fuller explanation.

What else do we know about the NII?

The NII are found in the nerve cells of the cortex and basal ganglia. Since cells in these areas of the brain are lost, this suggests that the NII are important in causing the selective nerve cell death.

The NII contain accumulations of the first part of the huntingtin protein, but they also contain another protein called **ubiquitin**. As its name implies, this protein is found in all cells of animals and plants. When it binds to proteins, they are marked for destruction by the cell. There are many reasons why a cell needs to turn over proteins, but the coming together of the first part of the abnormal huntingtin and ubiquitin in the NII to form clumps indicates that there is something wrong with this mechanism.

Are NII seen in other disorders?

The answer to this is 'yes'. Huntington's disease is not the only disorder to be characterized by an expansion of a polyglutamine repeat. A few other neurological disorders are caused by exactly the same mechanism, although of course the proteins involved are different from huntingtin. These other neurological disorders are also characterized by selective nerve cell death, but the pattern is specific for each of them. The discovery of NII in Huntington's disease prompted similar studies to be undertaken in the brains of patients with these other disorders, and, sure enough, NII have been found. This adds further weight to the idea that the NII are important to the understanding of selective nerve cell death in Huntington's disease and related disorders.

Are the NII causing the nerve cell death or are they a by-product of the main problem?

Although the NII are clearly important to understanding what is happening in Huntington's disease, it is not certain that they are the actual cause of the nerve cell death. A recent series of experiments, using brain cells grown in a laboratory, has tested some of the steps in the pathway. When abnormal huntingtin was modified so that it was transported back out of the nucleus, the nerve cells survived. This is consistent with the idea that abnormal huntingtin is transported into the nucleus and interacts there to produce nerve cell damage. Modifications were made to the ubiquitin (the other protein in the clumps) so that the NII did not form. In this experiment, which allowed abnormal huntingtin to enter the nucleus but prevented the formation of NII, the nerve cells still died—in fact, they died at a faster rate. The conclusion from these experiments was that it was not the NII which led directly to the nerve cell death. Instead, the abnormal huntingtin in the nucleus causes damage and the cell forms the NII as a way of protecting itself.

Conclusion

This chapter described two different possible themes to explain the selective nerve cell death. Neither explanation is complete in itself. Whilst it is not possible to provide a detailed explanation of the cause of the selective nerve cell death, considerable progress in understanding has occurred in the last few years.

In one theme the abnormal huntingtin somehow leads to abnormal energy production of some cells, which renders them more vulnerable to the toxic effects of chemical messengers in the brain. How the abnormal huntingtin leads to abnormal energy production is unclear.

In another theme, abnormal huntingtin enters the nucleus and damages the cells. As a consequence of this, the cells undergo premature programmed cell death. A marker for huntingtin entering the nucleus is the formation of NII.

It is important to understand the basic process in order to think about ways of developing effective treatments. These thoughts will be described in the next chapter.

8
Ideas for effective treatment of Huntington's disease

In writing this chapter I do not want to be too optimistic that effective treatment is around the corner and that all will be well in a few years time. Of course I would be delighted if this were to be the case. On the other hand, if Huntington's disease affects you or your relatives, it is important that ideas for effective treatment are being considered and that the research activity I described in the previous chapter is leading somewhere.

I also want to emphasize that there is a difference between effective treatment and a cure. If someone has a serious infection and is treated with appropriate antibiotics then the person can be restored to good health and is cured. On the other hand, if someone has a chronic condition, like diabetes, then giving them insulin is very effective treatment. The injections with insulin do not cure the underlying damage, which in this example is to cells in the pancreas.

A cure for Huntington's disease might involve getting rid of the abnormal huntingtin from the nerve cells of the brain. Whilst this might be wonderful, it is difficult to see how this could be achieved. More realistically, it would also be very valuable to develop a treatment which slowed the rate of selective nerve cell death: this would be an effective treatment.

Ideas based on the toxic model of Huntington's disease

The early animal models of Huntington's disease used toxic substances to mimic the selective nerve cell death. These experiments implicated the NMDA receptor as being important in the disease process. If drugs could be found which block the NMDA receptor without causing too many side-effects that might be a useful way forward. One such compound is **remacemide**. It is too early to say whether or not this is an effective treatment but trials are being conducted so there should be an answer to this question.

Treatments to address abnormal energy production

There is evidence from experiments that energy production is abnormal in cells and it is this which renders cells susceptible to damage. One way forward could be to use medicines which help overcome blocks to energy production in the cell. One such trial is under way, but again it will be some time before any definite information is known.

What about nerve cell transplants?

At first glance this seems a very radical solution to the problem. The idea is that fetal nerve cells have the potential to grow and develop. If fetal cells can be obtained then they could be implanted into the basal ganglia. The question arises as to whether they would then grow, make appropriate connections with other nerve cells, and effectively replace the nerve cells which have been lost. Such a programme raises all sorts of questions, but experiments in animal models of the disease have been promising.

At the moment it is not possible to request a fetal nerve cell transplant. It would be a mistake to rush into this type of experiment on humans unless certain conditions had been met. Some of these include: careful study of transplants in animals; careful study of volunteer patients so that the disease process is well documented in these patients before any procedure is attempted; and careful follow-up afterwards so that the effects of the transplant are understood. At this time, information from some animal studies is available but studies on volunteers have not been undertaken to an extent which allows any comment to be made.

What about trying to protect nerve cells from damage?

In animal models of the disease, injection of cells which secrete nerve growth factors helps to protect against toxic damage. Whether these experiments in animal models of the disease will lead to effective treatment is unclear. If this line of enquiry were to be successful then it might be possible to treat individuals with a positive predictive test result before significant nerve cell damage had occurred.

Conclusion

It is not possible to say very much about these ideas for treatment. As more is understood about the basic cause of the nerve cell death, so it will be possible to predict which treatment methods have the greatest chance of success.

9
Patients' organizations

Over the last few decades patient support groups have developed for many conditions. In some cases, these have become powerful charities in their own right. Any description of Huntington's disease would be incomplete without a discussion of the patients' organizations which can be a valuable source of information and support.

Marjorie Guthrie's role

One of the very first organizers of patients' groups was Marjorie Guthrie. She was the second wife of Woody Guthrie, the American folk singer. Woody had a colourful and extraordinary life which was captured in a biography written in 1980. In addition to describing the social conditions in America which helped shape Woody's songs, the biography also describes the effects of Huntington's disease on Woody and his family. In 1967, which also happened to be the year of Woody's death, Marjorie

Guthrie founded a Committee to Combat Huntington's Disease. From that time until her death in 1983 Marjorie Guthrie was a powerful advocate for Huntington's disease in America and internationally.

How did the patients' organization develop in the UK?

Whilst it is unfair to single out a specific story, it does serve as an illustration of how patients' organizations form and develop. The founder of the lay organization in the UK was Mauveen Jones. Mauveen's father had Huntington's disease as did other members of her family. In the summer of 1970 she read a newspaper article about Woody's son, Arlo Guthrie. Although the article was about folk music, Mauveen's attention was drawn to the paragraph about Arlo's father, Woody, dying of Huntington's disease. As a consequence, Mauveen wrote to Arlo, via the newspaper, and received a reply from Marjorie Guthrie enclosing her first newsletter. In the December of that year Mauveen read an article in another newspaper about an English family with Huntington's disease. This prompted her to write a letter to the newspaper inviting others with experience of this rare illness to contact her. This was the foundation of the 'United Kingdom Committee to Combat Huntington's Chorea' or 'Combat' for short. In due course similar organizations developed in Scotland and Northern Ireland. In more recent times the organization has changed its name to the 'Huntington's Disease Association' or HDA.

Origins of the World Federation of Neurology Huntington's Disease Research Group and the International Huntington Association

Professionals in the World Federation of Neurology (WFN) Huntington's Disease Research Group and lay members in the International Huntington Association meet together on alternate years. This has become a regular fixture for the international exchange of information between those affected by Huntington's disease in their families and researchers studying the condition. It may be worthwhile to record how these two groups started.

André Barbeau and a group of six doctors interested in Huntington's disease met in Montreal at a World Federation of Neurology Neurogenetics and Neuro-ophthalmology Congress in 1967. They resolved to meet every two years, and subsequent meetings have been held at different venues around the world. This origin explains the rather long title of World Federation of Neurology Huntington's Disease Research Group.

The first international meeting of patients' organizations occurred in 1974 when representatives from Canada and England met at the annual meeting of the American Huntington's disease organization. The Dutch lay organization was founded in April 1976 and Marjorie Guthrie was an invited speaker. One year later the WFN Huntington's Disease Research Group was due to meet in Lieden, Holland. The organizers arranged for a meeting of international lay societies to meet in the same building. At that time there were representatives from the USA, Canada, UK, Australia, Belgium, and Holland. Two years later the research group met in Oxford, and the patients' organization again arranged to meet in the same place at the same time. It was at that meeting, in 1979, that the IHA was officially formed. At the time of writing the most recent meeting of the two groups took place in Sydney Australia in 1997 and representatives were present from patients' organizations from 25 countries.

What is the role of a patients organization?

To some extent this varies from country to country and from organization to organization. Some of the aims of most organizations are:

- to disseminate information about Huntington's disease to families via newsletters and pamphlets;
- to disseminate knowledge of Huntington's disease to local doctors, social workers, nursing homes, and governments;
- to arrange or facilitate meetings of local groups;
- to raise funds to employ staff who will visit and support families;
- to raise funds to foster research;
- to raise funds to provide financial assistance to the membership.

Should you join the patients' organization?

This is obviously up to you. Some people like to join organizations whilst others do not. Given that

Huntington's disease is a rare disorder, some families benefit from knowing that they are not unique. Involvement can be simply at the level of reading newsletter, whereas others want to meet other families, attend lectures on the subject, and help with the fund-raising. At the very least you should be aware of the existence of the organizations so that it is possible to make contact in the future. A list of international addresses is given in the Appendix.

Appendix: Addresses of patients' organizations

AUSTRALIA

Australian Huntington's Disease Association
Post Box 178
2114 West Ryde
NSW
Australia
Tel: 61-2-9874 9777
Fax: 61-2-9874 9177

AUSTRIA

Östereichsche Huntington Hilfe
Hasnserstrasse 88/23
1160 Vienna
Austria
Tel: 43-1-4929 153

BELGIUM

Huntington Liga
Krijkelberg 1
B 3360 Leuven
Belgium
Tel: 32-16-452 759
Fax: 32-16-463 079

Ligue Huntington Francophone Belge
Rue De Brouckere 19
6150 Anderlues
Belgium
Tel: 32-87-675 408

BRAZIL

Dr Francisco Salzano
Departemento De Genetica
Instituto De Biociencias
Ufrgs
Caixa Postal 15053
91501-970 Porto Alegere Rs
Brazil
Tel: 55-51-316 6747
Fax: 55-51-319 3011
Email: Salzano@ifl.if.ufrgs.br

CANADA

Huntington Society of Canada
Box 1269
Cambridge, Ontario
N1R 7G6
Canada
Tel: 1-519-622 1002
Fax: 1-519-622 7370

Huntington Society of Quebec
4841 Rivard Street
Montreal
Quebec
N2J 2N7
Canada
Tel: 1-514-842 5740
Fax: 1-514-842 5961

CZECH REPUBLIC

**Spolecnost Pro Pomoc Pri
Huntingtonove Chorobe**
Dolni Brezany 153
25241 Dolni Brezany
Czech Republic
Tel: 42-2-2490 4261/2490 4269
Fax: 42-2-294 905

DENMARK

**Landsforeningen Mod
Huntington's Chorea**
Rosenvaenget 14
4270 Hong
Denmark
Tel: 45-5885 3003
Fax: 45-5885 0036

ECUADOR

Dr Nelson Penafiel-Revelo
Toledo 1233 Y Luis Cordero
Quito
Ecuador
Tel: 593-2-526 230
Fax: 593-2-503 575

FINLAND

**Huntington Association of
Finland**
Meriraumantie 21 As6
Sf 26200 Rauma
Finland
Tel: 358-2-821 1632
Fax: 358-2-822 404

FRANCE

Association Huntington France
42 44 Rue Du Chateau Des
Rentiers
75013 Paris France
Tel: 33-1-6986 9047
Fax: 33-1-6986 6050

GERMANY

Deutsche Huntington Hilfe
Postfach 281251
D47241 Duisburg
Germany
Tel: 49-203-22915
Fax: 49-203-22925

HUNGARY

Dr Bela Csala
Budal Nagy A.U. 14
7624 Pecs
Hungary
Tel: 36-72-314 344
Fax: 36-72-326 715

INDIA

Ms Mano Singh
K 18/7 Dlf Qutub Enclave Phase
11
35-66-77 Gurgaon Haryana
India
Tel C/O: 91-646-4544
Fax: 91-644-4221

IRELAND

**Huntington's Disease
Association of Ireland**
Carmichael House
North Brunswick Street
7 Dublin
Ireland
Tel: 353-1-872 1 303
Fax: 353-1-873 5737
Email: Ndai@indigo.ie

ISRAEL

Amita Huntington Israel
3 Lubezky Street
Gedera 70700
Israel

Tel: 972-8-859 8573
Fax: 972-2-670 8387
Email: Farkash@Netvision.Net.il

ITALY

Associazione Italiana Corea Di Huntington
Via L. Aristo 19
20145 Milano
Italy
Tel: 39-2-4801 5529
Fax: 39-2-239 4448

JAPAN

Dr Kaori Muto Yamamoto
The Health Care Science Institute
Akasaka Noa 5f 3-2-12 Akasaka
Minato-Ku
Tokyo 107
Japan
Tel: 81-3-5563-1791
Fax: 81-3-5563-1 795
Email: Nc-02@ppp.fastnet.or.jp

LITHUANIA

Prof. Valius Pauza M.D. Ph.D.
Head Neurological Department
& Clinic
Kaunas Medical Academy
Vice President of Lithuanian
Neurological Association
Mickeviciaus 9
Kaunas 3000
Lithuania
Tel: 370-7-792 627/733 849
Fax: 370-7-220 733

MALTA

Prof. Alfred Cuschiari
Dept of Anatomy, University of
Malta

Msida Msd 06
Malta
Tel: 356-336451
Fax: 356-336 450/ 356-319 527

MEXICO

Association Mexicana De La Enfermedad De Huntington A.C.
San Carlos #51
San Angel Inn
Mexico D.F. Cp 01060
Tel: 52-5-550 76 26

NETHERLANDS

Vereniging Van Huntington
Postbox 30470
2500 Gl Den Haag
Netherlands
Tel: 31-70-355 7414
Fax: 31-70-358 6174

NEW ZEALAND

Huntington's Disease Association of New Zealand
Postbox 78
Cust
North Canterbury
New Zealand
Tel: 64-3-3125 612
Fax: 64-4-232 5365

NORTHERN IRELAND

Huntington's Disease Association of Northern Ireland
Dept of Medical Genetics
Belfast, BT9 7AB
Northern Ireland
Tel: 353-232-653826

NORWAY

Landsforeningen For Huntington's Sykdom

Postbox 103
N 1415 Oppegard
Norway
Tel: 66-992477
Fax: 66-992477
Email:
Astrid.Jenssen@Vsit.V10.No

OMAN AND OTHER AFRICAN COUNTRIES

Dr Euan Scrimgeour
Dept of Medicine
College of Medicine
Sultan Qaboos University
Postbox 35
Al-Khod 123 Sultanate Of Oman
Tel: 968-513 333
Fax: 968-513 419

PAKISTAN

Huntington Disease Care & Cure Society Of Pakistan
2 Sawati Gate
Peshawar Cantt
Pakistan
Tel: 92-521-275 471
Fax: 92-521-273 900

PARAGUAY

Prof. Carlo Todisco
Dr Hassler
5738 C. Alas Paraguayas
Asuncion
Paraguay

POLAND

Prof. Jacek Zaremba
Institute Psychiatry/Neurology
1/9 Sobieskiego Str
02-957 Warsaw
Poland

Tel: 48-22-6426611 Ext 248
Fax: 48-22-6425375

RUSSIA

Huntington Association of Russia
Inst of Neurology Ac Science
Volokolamskoye Shosse 80
123367 Moscow
Russia
Tel: 7-95-490
2103/4902039/4902506
Fax: 7-95-490 2210

SCOTLAND

Scottish Huntington's Association
Thistle House 61 Main Road
Elderslie
Johnstone, PA5 9BA
Scotland
Tel: 44-1505-322245
Fax: 44-1505-382980

SLOVAKIA

Spolecnost Pre Pomoc Pri Huntingtonovej Chorobe V Slovenskej Republike
Oddelinie Lekarskej Genetiky
97517 Banska Bystrica
Slovakia
Tel: 42-88-71 3 380
Fax: 42-88-320 65

SOUTH AFRICA

Huntington's Society of South Africa
Postbox 44501
Claremont
Cape Town 7735
South Africa
Tel: 27-21 938 491 1

Fax: 27-21 7614 438
Email: Jschron@ilink.Nis.ZA

SPAIN

Association De Corea De Huntington Espanola
Fund Jimenez Diaz
Serv Neurologia
Avda Reyes Catolicos 2
28040 Madrid
Spain
Tel: 34-1-544 9008
Fax: 34-1-549 7381

SWEDEN

Huntington Foreningen 1 Sverige
C/0 Nhr
Postbox 3284
Kungsgatan 32
10365 Stockholm
Sweden
Tel: 46-8-140 320
Fax: 46-8-241 315/
46-8-677 010

SWITZERLAND

Schweizerische Huntington Vereinigung
Amtshausgasse 3a
Ch 3235 Erlach
Switzerland
Tel: 41-323-3381 383
Fax: 41-323-3881 383
Email: Mosdav@Micronas.Com

UNITED KINGDOM

Huntington's Disease Association
108 Battersea High Street
London, SW1 3HP
United Kingdom

Tel: 44-171-223 7000
Fax: 44-171-223 9489
Email: Headoffice@Hda.Org.Uk

UNITED STATES OF AMERICA

Huntington's Disease Society of America
140 West 22nd Street 6th Floor
New York
NY 10011
USA
Tel: 1-212-242 1968
Fax: 1-212-243 2443

OTHER COUNTRIES

Gerrit R. Dommerholt
International Development
Officer Iha
Callunahof 8
7217 St Harfsen
Netherlands
Tel: 31-573-431595
Fax: 31-70-358 61 74

OTHER ORGANIZATIONS

Foundation For The Care And Cure of Huntington's Disease Inc. (FCCHD)
Ms Liz Mueller
8 Jennifer Drive
Holmdel NJ 07733 USA
Tel: 908-739-5621

Hereditary Disease Foundation
1427 7th Street #22
Santa Monica
CA 90401 USA

Huntington's disease: the facts

Http://Ourworld.Compuserve.Co
m/Homepages/Hereditary Disease
Foundation/

**International Huntington
Association (IHA)**
Development Officer
Callunahof 8
7217 St Harfsen
Netherlands
Tel: 31-573-431595
Fax: 31-70-358 61 74

Index

Readers are also directed to the glossary of terms on pp. xiii–xviii

Index